My Child Is Sick!

Expert Advice for Managing Common Illnesses and Injuries

3RD EDITION

Barton D. Schmitt, MD, FAAP

American Academy of Pediatrics

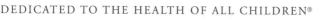

DEDICATED TO THE HEALTH OF ALL CHILDREN®

American Academy of Pediatrics Publishing Staff

Mary Lou White, *Chief Product and Services Officer/SVP, Membership, Marketing, and Publishing*
Mark Grimes, *Vice President, Publishing*
Kathryn Sparks, *Senior Editor, Consumer Publishing*
Shannan Martin, *Production Manager, Consumer Publications*
Amanda Helmholz, *Medical Copy Editor*
Sara Hoerdeman, *Marketing Manager, Consumer Products*

Published by the American Academy of Pediatrics
345 Park Blvd
Itasca, IL 60143
Telephone: 630/626-6000
Facsimile: 847/434-8000
www.aap.org

The American Academy of Pediatrics is an organization of 67,000 primary care pediatricians, pediatric medical subspecialists, and pediatric surgical specialists dedicated to the health, safety, and well-being of all infants, children, adolescents, and young adults.

The information contained in this publication should not be used as a substitute for the medical care and advice of your pediatrician. There may be variations in treatment that your pediatrician may recommend based on individual facts and circumstances.

Statements and opinions expressed are those of the authors and not necessarily those of the American Academy of Pediatrics.

Any websites, brand names, products, or manufacturers are mentioned for informational and identification purposes only and do not imply an endorsement by the American Academy of Pediatrics (AAP). The AAP is not responsible for the content of external resources. Information was current at the time of publication.

This publication has been developed by the American Academy of Pediatrics. The contributors are expert authorities in the field of pediatrics. No commercial involvement of any kind has been solicited or accepted in the development of the content of this publication. Disclosures: Dr Schmitt reports no conflicts of interest.

Every effort is made to keep *My Child Is Sick!* consistent with the most recent advice and information available from the American Academy of Pediatrics.

Author's disclaimer: This information is not intended to be a substitute for professional medical advice. It is provided for educational purposes only. You assume full responsibility for how you choose to use this information.

Your child's doctor has the final word. If your child's doctor tells you something that is different from what's in this book, follow your doctor's advice. Your doctor has the advantage of knowing you and your child and taking an actual history and performing a physical examination before making a decision.

You know your child better than anyone else. If you remain uncomfortable with your child's symptoms or condition after reading this book, please call your doctor or nurse for additional assistance. Finally, if you think your child has a life-threatening condition (such as struggling to breathe), always call 911 now.

Special discounts are available for bulk purchases of this publication.
Email Special Sales at nationalaccounts@aap.org for more information.

Printed in the United States of America

9-484/0922   1 2 3 4 5 6 7 8 9 10

CB0131

ISBN: 978-1-61002-616-1
eBook: 978-1-61002-619-2
EPUB: 978-1-61002-617-8

Cover design by Daniel Rembert

Publication design by Linda Diamond

Library of Congress Control Number: 2021922276

Praise for the First Edition of *My Child Is Sick!*

"An immensely helpful medical guide that won't just sit on the shelf . . . an excellent resource that will help all parents rest a little easier at night."—*Kirkus Reviews*, starred review

"This is a valuable and well-organized book that should be on the ready-reference shelf of every family home."—*Library Journal*

"Those desiring concise, practical guidance will appreciate the straightforward nature of this no-nonsense resource."—*Publishers Weekly*

"Helps parents and caregivers identify symptoms of everyday childhood maladies. . . . Thankfully, all information—including the detailed . . . Care Advice—is presented in clear checklist style. Such visual organization will be a blessing to parents, especially for those unavoidable moments of panic in the middle of the night."—*BookPage*

"*My Child Is Sick!* had guidance faster than I could google it. . . . It's a no-frills guide that doesn't mess around with anecdotes or fancy writing when all you want to know is how worried you should be."
—*The Tampa Tribune*

"It's a perfect back-to-school item for parents."—*Lincoln Journal Star*

"Chapters pertaining to the body part that 'hurts' offer easy-to-follow advice on how to treat ailments at home and when it's time to call the doctor."
—*Scholastic Parent & Child*

"*My Child Is Sick!* is a must-have for every parent, new or seasoned. Dr Schmitt's long-trusted content is written in a format that is easy to understand and answers many questions all parents have."—Suzanne Wells, MSN, RN, Manager, St. Louis Children's Hospital Answer Line, Past President, American Academy of Ambulatory Care Nursing

Equity, Diversity, and Inclusion Statement

The American Academy of Pediatrics is committed to principles of equity, diversity, and inclusion in its publishing program. Editorial boards, author selections, and author transitions (publication succession plans) are designed to include diverse voices that reflect society as a whole. Editor and author teams are encouraged to actively seek out diverse authors and reviewers at all stages of the editorial process. Publishing staff are committed to promoting equity, diversity, and inclusion in all aspects of publication writing, review, and production.

Contents

Part 6
Mouth or Throat Symptoms

Part 7
Lung or Breathing Symptoms

Part 8
Abdominal Symptoms

Part 9
Genital or Urinary Symptoms

Part 10
Arm or Leg Symptoms

Introduction

Most of the time your child is well—hungry at mealtime, sleeps soundly. Your family has fun together. The days fly by.

Then without warning, your child is sick or injured. You're uncertain what to do next. Should you call your child's doctor? Should you go to the ER? Can you treat your child at home? What's the current best advice for relieving your child's symptom?

That's why you have this book.

The first purpose of *My Child is Sick!* is to help you determine how sick your child is and if you need to call your child's doctor. The second purpose is to help you treat your child at home when it is safe to do so.

Here's what the book covers.

► The most common illnesses and injuries of childhood. At some point your child will develop most of these symptoms. You won't have to search through endless descriptions of uncommon conditions to find what you need.

► Decision checklists on when to call your child's doctor and when it's safe to treat your child at home. It teaches what symptoms are normal during the course of an illness or recovery from an injury. It also describes which symptoms are cause for concern and gives a specific time frame in which you need to call your child's doctor. About half the time, you can safely take care of your child at home without even calling your doctor.

► Specific, in-depth home care (treatment) advice for each symptom. You won't have to guess about the details of how to make your child feel better. And the advice is identical to that given by telephone nurses in most pediatric offices and hospital-based advice lines.

► Drug dosage charts for the most commonly used nonprescription medicines.

► Specific reassurance and facts to help you manage worrisome but nonserious symptoms.

► Finally, you are an important member of your child's health care team. Trust your parental instincts; they are a special safeguard for protecting your child. And never underestimate your common sense and potential to learn more about common illnesses and injuries. This book can empower you to provide optimal care for your sick child.

Using This Book

Select a Chapter

Choose the chapter that most closely matches your child's symptoms.

► If your child has more than one symptom, address the most serious symptom first. The most serious symptom is the symptom that could potentially cause the most harm to your child. (For example, for nosebleed and head injury together, use Chapter 5, Head Injury.) If you aren't sure which chapter to use, use more than one.

► Don't use Chapter 1, Fever, unless fever is your child's only symptom. If your child also has a cough, diarrhea, or another symptom, go to that chapter instead of fever.

► Choosing the appropriate symptom is very important because it leads you to the best information for your child's illness or injury.

Read the Chapter

Each chapter has 3 sections: **Definition, When to Call Your Doctor,** and **Care Advice.**

❶ Definition. Go to the selected chapter and read the *definition* to be sure it's a good fit for your child's problem. If not, consider related symptoms listed under the section *See Other Chapter If.*

❷ When to Call Your Doctor. Following the *Definition* section in each chapter, there is a decision section that helps you decide what action you should take. Below each response is a checklist of symptoms or reasons for taking that action. Read through these bulleted items. Read from top to bottom and don't skip any symptoms or reasons. The purpose of these is to help you determine the seriousness of your child's illness or injury. Once you have a positive symptom, stop reading and take the action suggested in the heading at the top of the list. This process is called *self-triage.*

❸ Care Advice. If your child has none of the Call Your Doctor symptoms, follow the home care advice listed in the final section. But watch your child carefully for any worsening or new symptoms. If your child's condition changes for the worse or you are uncomfortable with how your child looks or acts, call your child's doctor again.

Parent Responses: Decide What to Do and Do It

One of the purposes of this book is to help you determine how sick your child is. Then it is time to make a decision and act. By reading the *When to Call Your Doctor* section and using your common sense, you should be able to fit your child into 1 of the following 6 **When to Call Your Doctor** categories:

► Call 911 for an ambulance now.

► Go to an ER or urgent care center now.

► Call your child's doctor's office or a community nurse line for advice now.

► Call your child's doctor within 24 hours.

► Call your child's doctor during office hours.

► Take care of your sick child at home.

What you do depends on your child's symptoms and how sick your child looks. Here are some examples.

Call 911 Now for Life-threatening Emergencies Such As

► Breathing stopped, severe choking, severe trouble breathing, or face looks blue

► Can't wake up (in a coma)

► Having a seizure now

► Severe neck injury

► Severe bleeding and you can't stop it by pressing on the wound

Go to the ER Now for Serious Symptoms Such As

► Broken bones or other major injuries.

► Cuts that are split open and need stitches.

► Severe pain or crying that will not stop.

► Your child is acting confused, not alert, or out of it.

► Dehydration: No urine (pee) in over 8 hours, dark urine, very dry mouth, and no tears.

- Trouble breathing, fast breathing, wheezing, or retractions (ribs pulling in with each breath).

Call Your Child's Doctor's Office or a Community Nurse Line Now If

- You think your child might need to see a doctor, but you're not sure.

- Advice in this book told you to call.

- Your child's symptoms become worse.

- You have questions about refills, medicines, or vaccine shot reactions.

- Here's what will happen if you call: Nurses with special training will help you decide whether your child needs to see a doctor. Half the time, the nurse can tell you how to treat your child at home and save you a trip to the doctor.

- Summary: If you don't have an emergency, call a nurse for help.

Go to Your Child's Doctor's Office or Clinic If

- The phone nurse thinks your child needs to see a doctor.

- You're sure your child needs to see a doctor.

- Examples are ear infections, strep throat infections, and urinary tract infections.

- Make an appointment.

Take Care of Your Sick Child at Home Using This Book If

- Most infections caused by a virus can be safely treated at home.

- Examples are colds, coughs, flu, sore throats, sinus congestion, vomiting, diarrhea, and fevers.

- These viral infections are never helped by antibiotics.

- Your job is to keep your child comfortable. This book tells you how to do that.

- It will save you lots of travel time, waiting room time, and missed work.

PART 1

Fever Symptoms

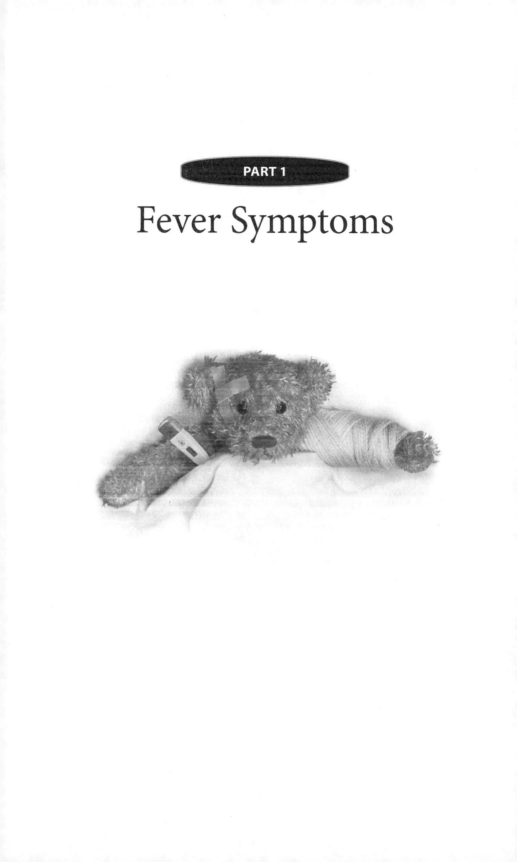

CHAPTER 1

Fever

Definition

► An abnormal high body temperature.

► Fever is the only symptom. Your child has a true fever if

• Rectal (bottom), ear, or forehead temperature: 100.4°F (38°C) or higher.

• Oral (mouth) temperature: 100°F (37.8°C) or higher.

• Under the arm (armpit) temperature: 99°F (37.2°C) or higher. If unsure, measure the temperature by another method to confirm fever.

► **Caution:** Ear temperatures are not accurate before 6 months of age.

► **Caution:** Forehead temperatures must be digital. Forehead strips are not accurate.

See Other Chapter If

► Other symptom is present with the fever; see that chapter. Examples are colds (Chapter 15), cough (Chapter 26), sore throat (Chapter 19), earache (Chapter 11), sinus pain or congestion (Chapter 16), diarrhea (Chapter 34), and vomiting (Chapters 35 and 36). (**Note:** If crying is the only other symptom, stay in this chapter.)

► See Chapter 57, Immunizations Reactions, if

• Fever started within 24 hours of getting a shot.

• Fever started 6 to 12 days after the measles shot.

• Fever started 17 to 28 days after the chickenpox shot.

Causes of Fever

► **Overview.** Almost all fevers are caused by a new infection. Viruses cause 10 times more infections than bacteria. The number of germs that causes an infection is in the hundreds. Only a few common ones will be listed.

► **Viral infections.** Colds, flu, and other viral infections are the most common cause. Fever may be the only symptom for the first 24 hours. The start of viral symptoms (runny nose, cough, loose stools) is often delayed. Roseola is the most extreme example. Fever may be the only symptom for 2 or 3 days. Then a rash appears.

- **Bacterial infections.** A bladder infection is the most common cause of silent fever in girls.
- **Sinus infection.** This is a complication of a cold. The main symptom is return of fever after it has been gone for a few days. Also, sinus congestion changes to sinus pain. Color of nasal discharge is not very helpful for making this diagnosis.
- **Vaccine fever.** Fever with most vaccines begins within 12 hours. It lasts 2 to 3 days. This is normal and harmless. It means the vaccine is working.
- **Newborn and infant fever (serious).** Fever that occurs during the first 3 months of life can be serious. All of these babies need to be seen as soon as possible. The fever may be due to sepsis (a bloodstream infection). Bacterial infections in this age group can worsen quickly and need rapid treatment.
- **Meningitis (very serious).** A bacterial infection of the membrane that covers the spinal cord and brain. Main symptoms are a stiff neck, headache, and confusion. Younger children are lethargic or so irritable that they can't be consoled. If not treated early, can cause brain damage.
- **Being overheated.** The fever is usually low-grade. Can occur during heat waves or from being overdressed. Temperature becomes normal in a few hours after moving to a cooler place. Can also occur during hard exercise. Fever goes away quickly with rest and drinking extra fluids.
- **Not due to teething.** Research shows that "getting teeth" does not cause fevers.

Fever and Crying

- Fever on its own shouldn't cause much crying.
- Frequent crying in a child with fever is caused by pain until proven otherwise.
- Hidden causes can be ear infections, kidney infections, sore throats, and meningitis.

Roseola: Classic Cause of Unexplained Fever in Young Children

- Most infants and children get roseola between 6 months and 3 years of age.
- **Cause:** *Human herpes virus 6.*
- **Classic feature:** 3 to 5 days of high fever without a rash or other symptoms.
- **Rash:** Pink, small, flat spots on the chest and stomach. Rash is the same on both sides of the body and then spreads to the face.
  - The rash starts 12 to 24 hours after the fever goes away.
  - The rash lasts 1 to 3 days.
  - Most children act mildly ill or even normal with roseola.

Normal Temperature Range

▶ **Rectal.** A reading of 98.6°F (37°C) is just the average rectal temperature. A normal low can be 96.8°F (36°C) in the morning. It can change to a high of 100.3°F (37.9°C) late in the day. This is a normal range.

▶ **Oral (mouth).** A reading of 97.6°F (36.5°C) is just the average oral temperature. A normal low can be 95.8°F (35.5°C) in the morning. It can change to a high of 99.9°F (37.7°C) late in the day. This is a normal range.

When to Call Your Doctor

Call 911 Now (Your Child May Need an Ambulance) If

▶ Not moving or too weak to stand.

▶ Can't wake up.

▶ Severe trouble breathing (struggling for each breath, can barely speak or cry).

▶ Purple or blood-colored spots or dots on the skin.

▶ You think your child has a life-threatening emergency.

Go to ER Now If

▶ You child has a stiff neck and can't touch chin to chest.

▶ **Age:** Younger than 1 year and soft spot bulging or swollen.

▶ Hard to wake up.

▶ Had a seizure with the fever.

▶ Not alert when awake (out of it).

▶ Acts or talks confused.

Call Your Doctor Now (Night or Day) If

▶ Trouble breathing, but not severe.

▶ Great trouble swallowing fluids or saliva (spit).

▶ **Age:** Younger than 12 weeks with any fever. (**Caution:** Do *not* give your baby any fever medicine before being seen.)

▶ Fever above 104°F (40°C).

▶ Shaking chills (shivering) lasting more than 30 minutes.

▶ Nonstop crying or cries when touched or moved.

- Won't move an arm or leg normally.

- Dehydration suspected (no urine in over 8 hours, dark urine, very dry mouth, and no tears).

- Burning or pain when passing urine.

- Weak immune system (such as sickle cell disease, HIV, cancer, organ transplant, or taking oral steroids).

- Your child looks or acts very sick.

- You think your child needs to be seen, and the problem is urgent.

Call Your Doctor Within 24 Hours If

- **Age:** 3 to 6 months with fever.

- **Age:** 6 to 24 months with fever that lasts more than 24 hours. There are no other symptoms (such as cough or diarrhea).

- Fever lasts more than 3 days.

- Fever returns after being gone for more than 24 hours.

- Recent travel outside the country to a high-risk area.

- You think your child needs to be seen, but the problem is not urgent.

Call Your Doctor During Weekday Office Hours If

- You have other questions or concerns.

Parent Care at Home If

- Fever with no other symptoms and your child acts mildly ill.

Care Advice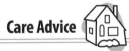

❶ What You Should Know About Fever

- Having a fever means your child has a new infection.

- It's most likely caused by a virus.

- You may not know the cause of fever until other symptoms develop. This may take 24 hours.

- Most fevers are good for sick children. They help the body fight infection.

- Use the ranges below to help put your child's level of fever into perspective.

  - **Low-grade fever:** Helpful, good range. Don't treat. 100°F to 102°F (37.8°C–39°C)

  - **Average fever:** Helpful. Treat if it causes discomfort. 102°F to 104°F (39°C–40°C)

  - **High fever:** Causes discomfort but is harmless. Always treat. Above 104°F (40°C)

  - **Very high fever:** Important to bring it down. Rare to go this high. Above 106°F (41.1°C)

  - **Dangerous fever:** Fever itself can be harmful. Above 108°F (42.2°C)

❷ Treatment for All Fevers: Extra Fluids

- Fluids alone can lower the fever. (**Reason:** Being well hydrated helps the body give off heat through the skin.)

- Offer your child water or other fluids by mouth. Cold fluids are better. Until 6 months old, only give extra formula or breast milk.

- For all children, dress in 1 layer of lightweight clothing, unless shivering. (**Reason:** Also helps heat loss from the skin.) **Caution:** If a baby younger than 1 year has a fever, never overdress or bundle up. (**Reason:** Babies can get over-heated more easily than older children.)

- For fevers 100°F to 102°F (37.8°C–39°C), fever medicines are rarely needed. Fevers of this level don't cause discomfort. They do help the body fight infection.

- **Exception:** If you feel your child also has pain, treat it.

❸ Fever Medicine

- Fevers need to be treated with medicine only if they cause discomfort. Most often, that means fevers above 102°F (39°C). Can use medicines for shivering (shaking chills). Shivering means the fever is going up.

- For fevers above 102°F (39°C), give an acetaminophen product (such as Tylenol) or ibuprofen product (such as Advil).

- **Goal of treatment:** Bring the temperature down to a comfortable level. Most often, fever medicine lowers the fever by 2°F to 3°F (1°C–1.5°C). It does not bring it down to normal. It takes 1 or 2 hours to see the effect.

- Do not use aspirin. (**Reason:** Risk of Reye syndrome, a rare but serious brain disease.)

- Do not use acetaminophen and ibuprofen together. (**Reason:** Not needed and a risk of giving too much.)

❹ Sponging With Lukewarm Water

- **Note:** Sponging is an option for high fevers, but not required. It is rarely needed.
- **When to use:** Fever above 104°F (40°C) and doesn't come down with fever medicine. Always give the fever medicine at least an hour to work before sponging.
- **How to sponge:** Use lukewarm water (85°F–90°F) (29.4°C–32.2°C). Sponge for 20 to 30 minutes.
- If your child shivers or becomes cold, stop sponging. Other option: You can also make the water warmer.
- **Caution:** Do not use rubbing alcohol. (**Reason:** Can cause a coma.)

❺ Return to School

- Your child can return to school or child care after the fever is gone. Your child should feel well enough to join in normal activities.

❻ What to Expect

- Most fevers with viral illnesses range between 101°F and 104°F (38.3°C and 40°C).
- They may last for 2 or 3 days.
- Most fevers are not harmful.

❼ Call Your Doctor If

- Your child looks or acts very sick.
- Any serious symptoms occur, such as trouble breathing.
- Fever rises above 104°F (40°C).
- Any fever occurs if your baby is younger than 12 weeks.
- Fever without other symptoms lasts more than 24 hours (if younger than 2 years).
- Fever lasts more than 3 days (72 hours).
- You think your child needs to be seen.
- Your child becomes worse.

Remember!
Contact your doctor if your child develops any of the **Call Your Doctor** symptoms.

CHAPTER 2

Fever: Myths Versus Facts

Definition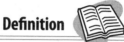

- ▶ Fever is a body temperature of 100.4°F (38°C) or higher.
- ▶ Fever is a symptom, not a disease.
- ▶ It happens whenever your child gets a new infection.
- ▶ Fever helps fight the infection by turning on the immune system.
- ▶ This topic reviews the known facts about fever.

Fever Phobia

- ▶ Parents often think fever will hurt their child. They worry and lose sleep when their child has a fever. This is called *fever phobia*.
- ▶ In fact, fevers are harmless. Here are some of the myths that cause fever phobia.

Fever Myths

- ▶ All fevers are bad for children.
- ▶ Fevers can cause brain damage.
- ▶ Fever can cause seizures in anyone.
- ▶ If the fever is high, the cause is serious.
- ▶ All fevers need to be treated with fever medicine.
- ▶ Without treatment, fevers will keep going up.
- ▶ If you can't "break the fever," the cause is serious.
- ▶ Treating the fever will make the infection go away faster.

Care Advice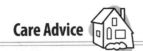

Facts About Fever That Every Parent Should Know

❶ Fevers are temperatures 100.4°F (38°C) or higher.

❷ Temperatures below 100.4°F (38°C) are normal. They are not a fever. The body temperature normally goes up during the day and comes down during the night. Don't make the mistake of treating normal temperatures.

❸ Fevers 100.4°F to 102°F (38°C–39°C) are low-grade fevers. Many doctors and nurses call them "good fevers."

❹ Fever helps the body fight infections. It turns on the body's immune system. Fever is a defense response found in all animals. Fevers between 100°F and 104°F (37.8°C and 40°C) actually help sick children get better.

❺ High fevers are 104°F (40°C) or higher. While we call them "high," they are not harmful.

❻ Most fevers with infections stay below 104°F (40°C). Reason: The brain has a thermostat that keeps the body at the best temperature to fight the germs. Temperatures sometimes go to 105°F (40.6°C), but that temperature is also harmless. The brain knows when the body is too hot.

❼ Fevers from infections don't cause brain damage. Only fevers above 108°F (42°C) can cause brain damage. Temperatures that high are very rare. They are caused by human error. An example would be a child left in a closed car during hot weather.

❽ Seizures triggered by fever are uncommon. Only 4% of children can have a seizure from fever. While these seizures are scary to watch, most stop within 2 minutes. And they don't cause any permanent harm, such as learning problems or seizures without fever.

❾ Most fevers with viral infections last 2 or 3 days. The fever will go away and not return once the body overpowers the virus. Most often, this is day 3 or 4. When using fever medicines, expect the fever to keep coming back after the medicine wears off. That's normal.

❿ If your child is well and feels warm to touch, they probably don't have a fever. Children can feel warm for many reasons. Examples are playing hard, crying hard, getting out of a warm bed, or hot weather. They are giving off heat. Their skin temperature should return to normal within 20 minutes after exercise.

⓫ **If your child acts sick and feels warm to touch, they probably have a fever.** If you want to be sure, take their temperature. But you don't need to keep taking it.

⓬ **Summary: Look at your child, not the thermometer.** How your child looks is what's important. The exact temperature number is not. If your child looks or acts very sick, the cause is more likely to be serious. But the level of fever tells us very little. Viruses and bacteria can both cause high fevers.

Treatment of Fever: When to Give Fever Medicines

❶ **Doctors and nurses don't always agree on when to treat fevers.** Here are some general guidelines.

❷ **Fevers need to be treated only if they cause discomfort.** Most fevers don't cause any discomfort until they go above 104°F (40°C). Discomfort at a lower fever is probably due to some pain (such as from a sore throat).

❸ **Start medicines for fevers only if higher than 102°F (39°C).** Remember that fevers are needed to fight the infection.

❹ **Treat fevers with one fever medicine.** Use either acetaminophen (such as Tylenol) or ibuprofen, in the correct dosage. Don't give both fever medicines together. **Reason:** It is not needed. Remember, fever is helping your child's body fight the infection.

❺ **With treatment, most fevers come down about 2°F (about 1°C).** They often don't come down to normal. That's fine. When the fever medicine wears off, expect the fever to go up again. That's also normal.

❻ **If your child's doctor tells you to treat fevers differently, follow their advice.**

❼ **Call Your Doctor If**

- You have other questions or concerns.

Summary

Keep in mind that fever is fighting off your child's infection. Fever is one of the good guys.

CHAPTER 3

Fever: How to Take the Temperature

Definition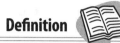

When Does Your Child Have a Fever?

▸ Rectal, forehead (temporal), or ear temperature: 100.4°F (38°C) or higher.

▸ Oral (mouth) temperature: 100°F (37.8°C) or higher.

▸ Under the arm (armpit) temperature: 99°F (37.2°C) or higher. If unsure, measure the temperature by another method to confirm fever.

▸ **Caution:** Ear temperatures are not accurate before 6 months of age.

Where to Take the Temperature

▸ Rectal temperatures are the most accurate. Forehead temperatures are the next most accurate. Oral and ear are also accurate if done properly. Temperatures taken in the armpit are the least accurate. Armpit temperatures are useful for screening at any age.

▸ **Age:** Younger than 3 months (90 days). An armpit temperature is the safest and is good for screening. If the armpit temperature is above 99°F (37.2°C), recheck it by using a rectal reading. (**Reason:** If young babies have a fever, they need to see a doctor now. New research shows that forehead temperatures may also be accurate in babies younger than 3 months.)

▸ **Age:** 3 months to 4 years. Rectal or electronic forehead temperatures are accurate. An ear thermometer can be used after 6 months of age. An armpit temperature is good for screening if it is taken correctly.

▸ **Age:** 5 years or older. Safe to take the temperature orally (by mouth). Ear and forehead thermometers are also good.

▸ Digital (electronic) thermometers are easily found in stores. They do not cost very much. They can be used for rectal, armpit, and oral temperatures. Most of them give an accurate temperature in 10 seconds or less. The American Academy of Pediatrics suggests you replace any glass thermometer with one of these products.

Rectal Temperature: How to Take It

▸ **Age:** Birth to 4 years.

▸ Have your baby or child lie stomach down on your lap. Another way is on the back with the legs pulled up to the chest.

▸ Put some petroleum jelly on the end of the thermometer and anus.

▸ Slide the thermometer gently into the anus no more than 1 in (2.5 cm). If your baby is younger than 6 months, put it in no more than ½ in (1.3 cm). That means until you can no longer see the silver tip. Be gentle. There should not be any resistance. If there is, stop.

▸ Hold your child still. Leave a digital thermometer in until it beeps (about 10 seconds).

▸ Your child has a fever if the rectal temperature is above 100.4°F (38°C).

Armpit Temperature: How to Take It

▸ **Age:** Any age for screening.

▸ Put the tip of the thermometer in an armpit. Make sure the armpit is dry.

▸ Close the armpit by holding the elbow against the chest. Do this until it beeps (about 10 seconds). The tip of the thermometer must stay covered by skin.

▸ Your child has a fever if the armpit temperature is above 99°F (37.2°C). If you have any doubt, take your child's temperature by rectum or forehead.

Oral Temperature: How to Take It

▸ **Age:** 4 years and older.

▸ If your child had a cold or hot drink, wait 30 minutes.

▸ Put the thermometer under one side of the tongue toward the back. It's important to put the tip in the right place.

▸ Have your child hold the thermometer with his lips and fingers, not teeth, to keep it in place. Keep the lips sealed until it beeps (about 10 seconds).

▸ Your child has a fever if the temperature is above 100°F (37.8°C).

Digital Pacifier Temperature: How to Take It

▸ **Age:** Birth to 1 year. Only good for screening. Requires the baby to suck on it, which is not always possible.

▸ Have your baby suck on the electronic pacifier until it beeps (about 10 seconds).

▸ Your baby has a fever if the pacifier temperature is above 100°F (37.8°C).

Ear Temperature: How to Take It

▶ **Age:** 6 months and older (not accurate before 6 months).

▶ This electronic thermometer reads the heat waves coming off the eardrum.

▶ A correct temperature depends on pulling the ear backward. Pull back and up if older than 1 year.

▶ Then aim the tip of the ear probe between the opposite eye and ear.

▶ Parents like this thermometer because it takes less than 2 seconds. It also does not need their child to cooperate. It does not cause any discomfort.

▶ **Caution:** Being outdoors on a cold day will cause a low reading. Your child needs to be inside for 15 minutes before you take the temperature. Earwax, ear infections, and ear tubes do not keep you from getting correct readings.

Forehead (Temporal Artery) Temperature: How to Take It

▶ **Age:** Any age.

▶ This electronic thermometer reads the heat waves coming off the temporal artery. This blood vessel runs across the forehead just below the skin.

▶ Place the sensor head at the center of the forehead.

▶ Slowly slide the thermometer across the forehead toward the top of the ear. Keep it in contact with the skin. (**Note:** Some newer forehead thermometers don't need to slide across the forehead. Follow the directions on how to take the temperature.)

▶ Stop when you reach the hairline.

▶ Read your child's temperature on the display screen.

▶ Used in more doctor's offices than any other thermometer.

▶ Parents like this thermometer because it takes less than 2 seconds. It also does not need their child to cooperate. It does not cause any discomfort.

▶ **Caution:** Forehead temperatures must be digital. Forehead strips are not accurate.

CHAPTER 4

Infection Exposure Questions and Chart

▶ This chapter includes information about the transmission of common infections. How long to stay out of school or child care is covered.

▶ **Incubation period:** Time it takes to start having symptoms after contact with infection.

▶ **Contagious period:** Time during which a sick child's disease can spread to others. Sometimes, children can return to school or child care before this period is over.

▶ **Infections that cannot be spread to others:** Many common bacterial infections are not spread to others. Examples are ear, sinus, bladder, or kidney infections. Most pneumonia in children also can't be passed to others, but there are a few exceptions. Your child's doctor will tell you for sure. Sexually transmitted infections are usually not spread to children. But, they can be spread if there is sexual contact or shared bathing.

Table 4.1. Infection Exposure

Disease	Incubation Period (days)	Contagious Period
Skin Infections/Rashes		
Chickenpox	10–21	2 days before rash begins until all sores have crusts (6–7 days)
Fifth disease (erythema infectiosum)	4–14	7 days before rash begins, until rash begins
Hand-foot-and-mouth disease	3–6	Onset of rash until fever gone. If widespread blisters, return after blisters are dry (6–7 days).
Impetigo (strep or staph)	2–5	Onset of sores until 24 hours on antibiotic
Lice	7	Onset of itch until 1 treatment
Measles	8–12	4 days before rash appears until 4 days after that
Roseola	9–10	Onset of fever until fever gone for 24 hours
Rubella (German measles)	14–21	7 days before rash appears until 5 days after that
Scabies	30–45	Onset of rash until 1 treatment
Scarlet fever	3–6	Onset of fever or rash until at least 12 hours on antibiotic and fever is gone
Shingles[a]	14–16	Onset of rash until all sores have crusts (7 days)[b]
Warts	30–180	Minimally contagious[c]

Table 4.1. Infection Exposure *(cont)*

Disease	Incubation Period (days)	Contagious Period
Respiratory Infections		
Bronchiolitis	4–6	Onset of cough until 7 days after that
Colds	2–5	Onset of runny nose until fever gone
Cold sores (herpes)	2–12	Depends on age[d]
Coughs or croup, viral	2–5	Onset of cough until fever gone
COVID-19	2–10	Onset of symptoms until fever is gone and at least 10 days have passed. Symptoms must be improving.
Influenza	1–2	Onset of symptoms until fever gone more than 24 hours
Sore throat, strep	2–5	Onset of sore throat until at least 12 hours on antibiotic and fever is gone
Sore throat, viral	2–5	Onset of sore throat until fever gone
Tuberculosis	6–24 months	Onset of tuberculosis until 2 weeks on drugs[e]
Whooping cough	7–10	Onset of runny nose until 5 days on antibiotic
Intestinal Infections		
Diarrhea, bacterial	1–5	Onset of diarrhea until stools are formed[f]
Diarrhea, *Giardia*	7–28	Onset of diarrhea until stools are formed[f]
Diarrhea, traveler's	1–6	Onset of diarrhea until stools are formed[f]
Diarrhea, viral (*Rotavirus*)	1–3	Onset of diarrhea until stools are formed[f]
Hepatitis A	14–50	2 weeks before jaundice begins until jaundice resolved (7 days)
Pinworms	21–28	Minimally contagious[c]
Vomiting, viral	2–5	Onset of vomiting until it stops
Other Infections		
Infectious mononucleosis	30–50	Onset of fever until fever gone (7 days)
Meningitis, bacterial	2–10	7 days before symptoms until 24 hours on intravenous antibiotics in hospital
Meningitis, viral	3–6	Onset of symptoms until 1–2 weeks after that
Mumps	12–25	5 days before swelling until swelling gone (7 days)
Pinkeye without pus, viral	1–5	Mild infection[c]
Pinkeye with pus, bacterial	2–7	Onset of pus until 1 day on antibiotic eyedrops

[a] Shingles is contagious but would cause chickenpox in exposed person, not shingles.
[b] No need to isolate if sores can be kept covered.
[c] Staying home is unnecessary.
[d] Younger than 6 years: Until cold sores are dry (4–5 days). No isolation if sores are on part of body that can be covered. Older than 6 years: No isolation necessary if beyond touching or picking stage.
[e] Most childhood tuberculosis is not contagious.
[f] Stay home until fever is gone, diarrhea is mild, blood and mucus are gone, and toilet-trained child has control over loose stools. *Shigella* and *E coli* 0157 require extra precautions. Consult your child's doctor regarding attendance restrictions.

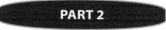
PART 2

Head or Brain Symptoms

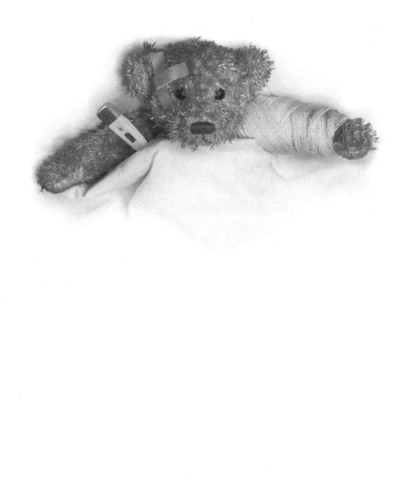

CHAPTER 5

Head Injury

Definition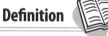

- ▶ Injuries to the head.

- ▶ Includes the scalp, skull, and brain.

Types of Head Injuries

- ▶ **Scalp injury:** Most head injuries damage only the scalp. Examples are a cut, scrape, or bruise, or swelling. It is common for children to fall and hit their head while growing up. This is especially common when a child is learning to walk. Big lumps (bruises) can occur with minor injuries. This is because there is a large blood supply to the scalp. For the same reason, small cuts on the head may bleed a lot. Bruises on the forehead sometimes cause black eyes 1 to 3 days later. This is caused by blood settling downward by gravity. (**Note:** Swelling of the scalp does not mean there is any swelling of the brain. The scalp and brain are not connected. They are separated by the skull bone.)

- ▶ **Skull fracture:** Only 1% to 2% of children with head injuries will get a skull fracture. Most often, there are no other symptoms except for a headache. The headache occurs at the site where the head was hit. Most skull fractures occur without any injury to the brain and heal easily.

- ▶ **Concussion:** A concussion is a type of brain injury. It causes a change in how the brain works for a short time. It is usually caused by a sudden blow or jolt to the head. Most children bump or hit their heads without causing a concussion. Most common signs are a brief period of confusion or memory loss. This happens after the injury. Other signs of a concussion can include a headache or vomiting. Dizziness or acting dazed can also be signs. A person does not need to be knocked out to have had a concussion. Following a concussion, some children have ongoing symptoms. These can include headaches, dizziness, or thinking difficulties. School problems or emotional changes can occur. These symptoms can last for several weeks.

- Brain injuries (serious) are uncommon. They include bleeding, bruises, or swelling within the brain. These are recognized by the following symptoms:
  - Hard to wake up or keep awake.
  - Acts or talks confused.
  - Slurred speech.
  - Weakness of arms or legs.
  - Walking is not steady.
- These symptoms are an emergency. If they happen, call 911.

Concussion Treatment

- Treating a concussion requires both physical and brain rest.
- Brain rest means a gradual return to full studying and school attendance.
- Physical rest means a gradual return to normal activity, work, and gym class.
- If symptoms occur (such as headache), your child needs to return to the previous level of physical and mental activity. In 24 hours, your child can try again to take it to the next level.
- Athletes involved in sports need to have a stepwise plan for "return to play." Progressing through stages should be supervised by a doctor or athletic trainer.
- Athletes of middle school age and older should take a preseason baseline cognitive function test. If a concussion occurs, this test may be repeated to see that the memory and reaction time have returned to normal before being released to return to play.

Pain Scale

- **Mild:** Your child feels pain and tells you about it. But, the pain does not keep your child from doing any normal activities. School, play, and sleep are not changed.
- **Moderate:** The pain keeps your child from participating in normal activities. It may wake your child up from sleep.
- **Severe:** The pain is very bad. It keeps your child from participating in all normal activities.

First Aid for Bleeding

- Put a gauze pad or clean cloth on top of the wound.
- Press down firmly on the place that is bleeding.

- This is called *direct pressure*. It is the best way to stop bleeding.
- Keep using pressure until the bleeding stops.
- If bleeding does not stop, press on a slightly different spot.

First Aid for Suspected Spinal Cord Injury

- Do not move your child until a spinal board is put on by paramedics.

When to Call Your Doctor

Call 911 Now (Your Child May Need an Ambulance) If

- Seizure occurred.
- Knocked out for more than 1 minute.
- Not moving neck normally. (**Caution:** Protect the neck from any movement.)
- Hard to wake up.
- Acts or talks confused or slurred speech present now.
- Walking not steady or weakness of arms/legs present now.
- Major bleeding that can't be stopped.
- You think your child has a life-threatening emergency.

Go to ER Now If

- Mild concussion suspected (awake but not alert, not focused, or slow to respond).
- Neck pain after head injury.
- Knocked out for less than 1 minute.
- Had confused talking, slurred speech, unsteady walking, or weakness of arms/ legs but fine now.
- Blurred vision lasted more than 5 minutes.
- Injury caused by high speed (car crash).
- Vomited 2 or more times.
- Severe headache or crying that won't stop.
- Can't remember what happened or store new memories.
- Large, deep cut that will need many stitches.

Call Your Doctor Now (Night or Day) If

▶ **Age:** Younger than 1 year.

▶ Skin is split open or gaping and may need stitches.

▶ Bleeding won't stop after 10 minutes of direct pressure.

▶ Large swelling (larger than 1 in or 2.5 cm).

▶ Large dent in skull.

▶ Blow from hard object (such as a golf club).

▶ Fall from a dangerous height.

▶ You think your child has a serious injury.

▶ You think your child needs to be seen, and the problem is urgent.

Call Your Doctor Within 24 Hours If

▶ Headache lasts more than 24 hours.

▶ You think your child needs to be seen, but the problem is not urgent.

Call Your Doctor During Weekday Office Hours If

▶ Dirty cut and no tetanus shot in more than 5 years.

▶ Clean cut and no tetanus shot in more than 10 years.

▶ You have other questions or concerns.

Parent Care at Home If

▶ Minor head injury.

Care Advice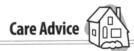

❶ What You Should Know About Mild Head Injuries

■ Most head injuries cause only a swelling or bruise to the scalp.

■ The main symptom is pain.

■ Swelling of the scalp does not mean there is any swelling of the brain. The scalp and brain are not connected. They are separated by the skull bone.

■ The skull bone protects the brain from getting injured.

■ Big lumps or bruising can occur with minor injuries to the scalp. This is normal. (**Reason:** The scalp has a large blood supply.)

- A concussion is a brain injury. Most of those also turn out fine.
- Following is some care advice that should help.

❷ Wound Care

- If there is a scrape or cut, wash it off with soap and water.
- For any bleeding, put direct pressure on the wound. Use a gauze pad or clean cloth. Press for 10 minutes or until the bleeding has stopped.

❸ Cold Pack for Swelling

- Use a cold pack or ice bag wrapped in a wet cloth. Put it on any swelling. Do this for 20 minutes.
- **Reason:** Prevents big lumps ("goose eggs"). Also, helps with the pain.
- Repeat in 1 hour and then as needed.

❹ Watch Your Child Closely for 2 Hours

- Watch your child closely during the first 2 hours after the injury.
- Have your child lie down and rest until all symptoms have cleared. (**Note:** Mild headache, mild dizziness, and nausea are common.)
- Allow your child to sleep if he wants to, but keep him nearby.
- Wake him up after 2 hours of sleeping. Check that he is alert and knows who you are. Also, check that he can talk and walk normally.

❺ Diet: Start With Clear Fluids

- Offer only clear fluids to drink, in case he vomits.
- Allow a regular diet after 2 hours.
- **Exception:** Babies can continue breastfeeding or formula.

❻ Pain Medicine

- To help with the pain, give an acetaminophen product (such as Tylenol). Another choice is an ibuprofen product (such as Advil). Use as needed.
- **Exception:** Do not give until 2 hours have passed since injury without any vomiting.
- **Caution:** Never give aspirin to children and teens. (**Reason:** Always increases risk of bleeding.)

❼ Special Precautions for 1 Night

- Mainly, sleep in the same room as your child during the night.

- **Reason:** If a problem occurs, you will recognize it if you are close by. Problems include a bad headache, vomiting, or confusion. Also, look for any change in your child's normal behavior.

- **Option:** If you are worried, wake your child once during the night. Check how he walks and talks.

- After 24 hours, return to a normal sleep routine.

❽ What to Expect

- Most head trauma causes only a scalp injury.

- Headache usually clears in 24 hours.

- Scalp pain at the site of impact may last 3 days.

- Swelling may take a week to go away.

❾ Call Your Doctor If

- Pain or crying becomes severe.

- Vomits 2 or more times.

- Your child becomes hard to wake up or confused.

- Walking or talking is not normal.

- Headache lasts more than 24 hours.

- You think your child needs to be seen.

- Your child becomes worse.

Remember!
Contact your doctor if your child develops any of the **Call Your Doctor** symptoms.

CHAPTER 6

Headache

Definition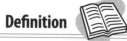

- ▶ Pain or discomfort of the head.
- ▶ This includes the forehead to the back of the head.
- ▶ Not caused by a head injury.

See Other Chapter If

- ▶ Head injury occurred within the last 3 days. See Chapter 5, Head Injury.
- ▶ Pain is around the eye or cheekbone. See Chapter 16, Sinus Pain or Congestion.

Causes of Acute Headaches

- ▶ **Viral illnesses.** Most acute headaches are part of a viral illness. Flu is a common example. These headaches may relate to the level of fever. Most often, they last a few days.
- ▶ **Hunger headaches.** About 30% of people get a headache when they are hungry. It goes away within 30 minutes of eating something.
- ▶ **Common harmless causes.** Hard exercise, bright sunlight, blowing a wind instrument, and gum chewing have been reported. So has severe coughing. Ice-cream headaches are triggered by any icy food or drink. The worst pain is between the eyes (bridge of the nose).
- ▶ **Head injury.** Most just cause a scalp injury. This leads to a painful spot on the scalp for a few days. Severe, deeper, or entire-head pain needs to be seen.
- ▶ **Frontal sinus infection.** Can cause a headache on the forehead just above the eyebrow. Other symptoms are nasal congestion and postnasal drip. Rare before 10 years of age. (**Reason:** The frontal sinus is not yet formed. Other sinus infections cause face pain, not headaches.)
- ▶ **Meningitis (very serious).** A bacterial infection of the membrane that covers the spinal cord and brain. Main symptoms are a stiff neck, headache, confusion, and fever. Younger children are lethargic or so irritable that they can't be consoled. If not treated early, can cause brain damage or death.

Causes of Recurrent Headaches

► **Tension headaches.** Most common type of frequent headaches. Tension headaches give a feeling of tightness around the head. Neck muscles also become sore and tight. Tension headaches can be caused by staying in one position for a long time. This can happen when reading or using a computer. Other children get tension headaches as a reaction to stress or worry. Examples of possible triggers are pressure for better grades or family arguments.

► **Migraines.** Severe, very painful headaches that keep your child from participating in normal activities. They are throbbing and often occur on just one side. Symptoms have a sudden onset and offset. Vomiting or nausea is present in 80% of cases. Lights and sound make them worse. Most children want to lie down in a dark, quiet room. Migraines most often run in the family (genetic).

► **School avoidance.** Headaches that mainly occur in the morning on school days. They keep the child from going to school. The headaches are real and due to a low pain threshold.

► **Rebound headaches.** Caused by overuse of pain medicines in high doses. Most often happens with over-the-counter medicines. Caffeine is present in some pain medicines and may play a role. Treatment is taking pain medicines at the correct dosage.

► **Vision headaches.** Poor vision and straining to see the blackboard can cause eye pain. Sometimes, it can also cause a muscle tension headache. Getting glasses rarely solves a headache problem that doesn't also have associated eye pain.

Pain Scale

► **Mild:** Your child feels pain and tells you about it. But, the pain does not keep your child from doing any normal activities. School, play, and sleep are not changed.

► **Moderate:** The pain keeps your child from doing some normal activities. It may wake your child up from sleep.

► **Severe:** The pain is very bad. It keeps your child from doing all normal activities.

When to Call Your Doctor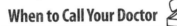

Call 911 Now (Your Child May Need an Ambulance) If

► Hard to wake up or passed out.

► Acts or talks confused.

▶ Weakness of arm or leg on one side of the body.

▶ You think your child has a life-threatening emergency.

Go to ER Now If

▶ Walking not steady.

▶ Stiff neck and can't touch chin to chest.

▶ Severe, constant pain (child not able to move or do anything).

▶ Severe migraine that persists after migraine medicine and going to sleep.

Call Your Doctor Now (Night or Day) If

▶ Vomiting.

▶ Blurred vision or seeing double.

▶ Your child looks or acts very sick.

▶ You think your child needs to be seen, and the problem is urgent.

Call Your Doctor Within 24 Hours If

▶ Fever.

▶ Sinus pain (not just congestion) of the forehead.

▶ Swelling around the eye with pain.

▶ You think your child needs to be seen, but the problem is not urgent.

Call Your Doctor During Weekday Office Hours If

▶ Headache without other symptoms lasts more than 24 hours.

▶ Migraine suspected, but never diagnosed.

▶ Sore throat lasts more than 48 hours.

▶ Any headache lasts more than 3 days.

▶ Headaches are a frequent problem.

▶ You have other questions or concerns.

Parent Care at Home If

▶ Mild headache.

▶ Migraine, just like past ones.

Care Advice

Treatment for Mild Headache

❶ What You Should Know About Mild Headaches

- Headaches are very common with some viral illnesses. Most often, these will go away in 2 or 3 days.
- Unexplained headaches can occur in children, just as they do in adults. They usually pass in a few hours or last up to a day.
- Most recurrent headaches that can occur in anyone are tension headaches.
- Most headaches (including tension headaches) are helped by the following measures:

❷ Pain Medicine

- To help with pain, give an acetaminophen product (such as Tylenol).
- Another choice is an ibuprofen product (such as Advil).
- Use as needed.
- Headaches due to fever are also helped by bringing the fever down.

❸ Food May Help

- Give fruit juice or food if your child is hungry.
- If your child hasn't eaten in more than 4 hours, offer some food.
- **Reason:** Skipping a meal can cause a headache in many children.

❹ Lie Down and Rest

- Lie down in a quiet place and relax until feeling better.

❺ Cold Pack for Pain

- Put a cold pack or cold, wet washcloth on the forehead.
- Do this for 20 minutes. Repeat as needed.

❻ Stretch Neck Muscles

- Stretch and rub any tight neck muscles.

❼ Tension Headache Prevention

- If something bothers your child, help her talk about it. Help her get it off her mind.

- Teach your child to take breaks when she is doing schoolwork. Help your child relax during these breaks.

- Teach your child the importance of getting enough sleep.

- Some children may feel pressure to achieve more. This may cause headaches. If this is the case with your child, help her find a better balance.

- **Caution:** Frequent headaches are often caused by too much stress or worry. To be sure, schedule a medical checkup for your child first.

❽ Call Your Doctor If

- Headache becomes severe.

- Vomiting occurs.

- Headache without other symptoms lasts more than 24 hours.

- Headache lasts more than 3 days.

- You think your child needs to be seen.

- Your child becomes worse.

Treatment for Migraine

❶ What You Should Know About Migraines

- This headache is like the migraines that your child has had before. If not, see your doctor.

- The sooner a migraine is treated, the more likely the treatment will work.

- Often the most helpful treatment is going to sleep.

- Here is some care advice that should help.

❷ Migraine Medicine

- If your child's doctor has prescribed a medicine for migraines, use it as directed. Give it as soon as the migraine starts.

- If not, you can use ibuprofen (such as Advil). It is the best over-the-counter drug for migraines. Give it now. Repeat in 6 hours if needed.

❸ Try to Sleep

- Have your child lie down in a dark, quiet place and try to sleep.

- People with a migraine often wake up from sleep with their migraine gone.

❹ Prevention of Migraines

- Drink lots of fluids.

- Don't skip meals.

- Get enough sleep each night.

❺ What to Expect

- With treatment, migraines usually go away in 2 to 6 hours.

- Most people with migraines get 3 or 4 per year.

❻ Return to School

- Children with a true migraine are not able to stay in school.

- Children with migraines also commonly get tension headaches. For those, they should take a pain medicine and go to school.

❼ Call Your Doctor If

- Headache becomes much worse than past migraines.

- Headache lasts longer than past migraines.

- You think your child needs to be seen.

Remember!
Contact your doctor if your child develops any of the **Call Your Doctor** symptoms.

CHAPTER 7

Crying Child

Definition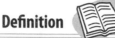

▶ A child older than 3 months is crying and you don't know why.

▶ Your child is too young to tell you why. (**Age:** Most of these children are younger than 2 years.)

▶ Crying is the only symptom.

See Other Chapter If

▶ Fever (Chapter 1) or any symptom of illness (such as cough [Chapter 26]). See table of contents.

▶ Crying from an injury. See Chapter 5, Head Injury; Chapter 40, Arm Injury; or Chapter 42, Leg Injury.

Causes of Unexplained Crying

▶ **New illness.** Coming down with an illness is the main physical cause. Young children cry about being sick, even if they don't have any pain.

▶ **Physical pain.** Painful causes include earache, sore throat, mouth ulcers, or a raw diaper rash. A sore on the penis or constipation may also cause pain or crying.

▶ **Behavioral causes.** Most crying means the child is upset about something. Crying can occur when a young child is separated from his parents. Other examples are crying with tantrums or when overtired. This chapter also covers crying caused by sleep problems. (Crying almost always occurs during retraining programs for bad sleep habits.) Some preverbal children cry any time they want something.

▶ **Hunger.** After the early months, most parents can recognize hunger and feed their child. If they don't, their child may cry.

▶ **Cold medicines.** Drugs like Sudafed can also cause crying. (**Note:** The US Food and Drug Administration does not advise cough and cold medicines for babies and children younger than 6 years.)

Myths About Causes of Crying

▶ **Not due to teething.** Teething may cause some babies to be fussy. But, in general, it does not cause crying.

▶ **Not due to gas.** Gas passing through normal intestines does not cause pain or crying.

When to Call Your Doctor

Call 911 Now (Your Child May Need an Ambulance) If

▶ Not moving or very weak.

▶ You think your child has a life-threatening emergency.

Go to ER Now If

▶ Stiff neck (can't touch chin to chest).

▶ Bulging soft spot.

▶ Swollen scrotum or groin.

▶ Won't move one arm or leg normally.

▶ Cries when touched or moved.

▶ Screaming and can't be consoled.

▶ Not alert when awake (out of it).

Call Your Doctor Now (Night or Day) If

▶ Could be an injury.

▶ Nonstop crying lasts more than 2 hours. (Your child can't be consoled after using this chapter's Care Advice.)

▶ You are afraid someone might hurt or shake your child.

▶ Will not drink or drinks very little for more than 8 hours.

▶ Your child looks or acts very sick.

▶ You think your child needs to be seen, and the problem is urgent.

Call Your Doctor Within 24 Hours If

▶ You think pain (such as an earache) is causing the crying.

▶ Crying but can be consoled. Cause of crying is not clear.

▶ You think your child needs to be seen, but the problem is not urgent.

Call Your Doctor During Weekday Office Hours If

► Mild, off-and-on fussiness without a cause lasts more than 2 days.

► Crying is a frequent problem.

► You have other questions or concerns.

Parent Care at Home If

► Mild fussiness without a cause is present fewer than 2 days.

► Normal protest crying.

► Tantrum crying.

► Sleep problem crying.

Care Advice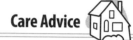

Mild Fussiness of Unknown Cause

❶ What You Should Know

■ Your child is crying and fussing more than normal. But, if acting normal when not crying, the cause is probably not serious.

■ He could be coming down with an illness. Most often, that will become clear in a day or so.

■ He could be reacting to some changes in your home or child care setting. See if you can come up with some ideas.

■ At times, children can also go through a "clingy phase" without a reason.

■ If the crying stops with comforting, it's not serious.

■ Here is some care advice that should help.

❷ Comfort Your Child

■ Try to comfort your child by holding, rocking, or massaging him.

■ Talk in a quiet, calm voice.

❸ Undress Your Child and Check the Skin

■ Sometimes, part of the clothing is too tight. Loosen it.

■ Also, check the skin for redness or swelling (such as an insect bite). Include fingers and toes.

❹ Stop Any Over-the-counter Medicines

- If your child is taking a cough or cold medicine, stop giving it.
- The crying should stop within 4 hours.
- Allergy medicine like Benadryl can cause screaming in a small number of children. Also, may cause some children to be more fussy than normal.
- Drugs that reduce congestion (like Sudafed) can cause crying.
- The US Food and Drug Administration does not approve any of these drugs for babies and children younger than 6 years.

❺ Sleep or Take a Nap

- If your child is tired, put him to bed.
- If he needs to be held, hold him quietly in your arms. Sometimes, lying next to him will comfort him.
- Some overtired infants need to fuss themselves to sleep.

❻ Warning: Never Shake a Baby

- It can cause bleeding on the brain. Severe brain damage can happen in a few seconds.
- Never leave your baby with someone who is too young, or has a bad temper.
- If you are frustrated, put your baby down in a safe place.
- Call or ask a friend or relative for help.
- Take a break until you calm down.

❼ What to Expect

- Most fussiness with illnesses goes away when the illness does.
- Fussiness may be due to family stress or change (such as new child care). Such fussiness lasts less than 1 week.

❽ Call Your Doctor If

- Nonstop crying lasts more than 2 hours.
- Crying with an illness gets worse.
- Mild crying lasts more than 2 days.
- You think your child needs to be seen.
- Your child becomes worse.

Normal Protest Crying

❶ What You Should Know

- Normal children cry when they don't get their way.
- Normal children cry when you make changes in their routines.
- Crying is how young children communicate in the first years of life.
- Crying can mean, "I don't want to."
- This is called *normal protest crying* and is not harmful.
- Do not assume that crying means pain.

❷ Call Your Doctor If

- Crying becomes worse.
- Your child does not improve with this advice.
- You have other questions or concerns.

Tantrum Crying

❶ What You Should Know

- Crying is the most common symptom of a tantrum.
- Tantrums occur when your child is angry or trying to get his way.
- This is likely the cause of crying if it occurs at these times.
- All kids have some tantrums, starting at about 9 months of age.

❷ Tips for Dealing With Tantrums

- Ignore most tantrums (such as your child wanting something he doesn't need).
- Don't give your child an audience. Leave the room.
- For tantrums from frustration (such as when something doesn't work), help your child.
- For tantrums that involve hitting or throwing objects, put your child in time-out. Leave him there until he calms down.
- Don't give in to tantrums. No means no.
- Be a good role model. Do not yell or scream at others (adult tantrums).

❸ Call Your Doctor If

- Crying becomes worse.
- Your child does not improve with this advice.
- You have other questions or concerns.

Sleep Problem Crying

❶ What You Should Know

- Sleep problems can cause crying. Recognize this if most of your child's crying occurs in his crib or bed, mainly when you put him down for naps and at night. Also, consider it a sleep problem if your child acts normal during the daytime.
- Sleep problems are common in childhood.

❷ Tips for Treating the Sleep Problem

- Retrain your child to be a good sleeper at bedtime and naptime.
- Place your child in the crib "sleepy but awake."
- Once your child is placed in the crib, don't take your child out again.
- If needed, visit your child every 10 minutes or so until he is asleep. (Exception: Each visit restarts the crying.)
- For waking at night, for now it's fine to hold your child until calm.
- Do all of this in a loving way with a calm voice.
- Never feed your child to get him/her to fall asleep. Always stop before asleep.
- Never sleep in the same bed with your child.

❸ Call Your Doctor If

- Crying becomes worse.
- Your child does not improve with this advice.
- You have other questions or concerns.

Remember!
Contact your doctor if your child develops any of the **Call Your Doctor** symptoms.

PART 3

Eye Symptoms

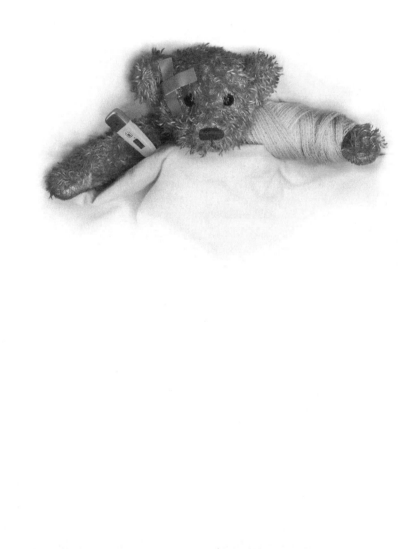

CHAPTER 8

Eye, Red Without Pus

Definition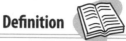

- ▶ Red or pink color of the white of the eye without any pus.
- ▶ The eye looks irritated.
- ▶ May have increased tears (a watery eye).
- ▶ Puffy eyelid (mildly swollen).
- ▶ No pus or yellow discharge.
- ▶ Not caused by an eye injury.

See Other Chapter If

- ▶ Yellow or green pus is in the eye. See Chapter 9, Eye, Pus or Discharge.
- ▶ Main symptom is itchy eyes. See Chapter 10, Eye Allergy.

Causes of Pinkeye (*Red Eye*)

- ▶ **Pinkeye defined.** When the white of the eye becomes pink or red, it's called *pinkeye*. *Conjunctivitis* is the medical name for pinkeye. The conjunctiva is the membrane that covers the white of the eye. It becomes pink or red when it is infected or irritated. Pinkeye (*conjunctivitis*) has many causes.

  - • **Viral conjunctivitis** is the main cause of pink or red eyes without pus. Most often, it is part of a cold.

  - • **Bacterial conjunctivitis.** Pinkeye plus the eyelids are stuck together with pus. Most likely, this is a secondary infection of a viral conjunctivitis.

  - • **Allergic conjunctivitis** from pollens. Most children with eye allergies also have nasal allergies (hay fever). Symptoms include sneezing and clear nasal discharge.

  - • **Irritant conjunctivitis** from sunscreen, soap, chlorine in pool water, smoke, or smog. Irritants can also be transferred by touching the eye with dirty fingers. Irritants can sometimes include food or plant resins.

- **Contact lens conjunctivitis.** Caused by poor use of disinfecting solution or keeping lenses in overnight.

- **Rebound conjunctivitis from vasoconstrictor eyedrops abuse.** Usually occurs in teen girls who use daily over-the-counter eyedrops to remove mild redness. After the medicine wears off, the blood vessels become larger than they were to begin with.

- **Foreign body (object).** If only one side has pinkeye, an object in the eye must be considered.

- **Palpebral cellulitis (serious).** A bacterial infection of the eyelids and skin around them. Causes the lids to be very red and swollen.

When to Call Your Doctor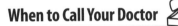

Call Your Doctor Now (Night or Day) If

▶ Eyelid is very red or very swollen.

▶ Nonstop tears or blinking.

▶ Vision is blurred.

▶ Eye pain that's more than mild.

▶ You child needs to turn away from any light.

▶ **Age:** Younger than 12 weeks with fever. (**Caution:** Do *not* give your baby any fever medicine before being seen by a doctor.)

▶ Your child looks or acts very sick.

▶ You think your child needs to be seen, and the problem is urgent.

Call Your Doctor Within 24 Hours If

▶ Only 1 eye is red and redness lasts more than 24 hours.

▶ Fever lasts more than 3 days.

▶ Fever returns after being gone for more than 24 hours.

▶ You think your child needs to be seen, but the problem is not urgent.

Call Your Doctor During Weekday Office Hours If

▶ **Age:** Younger than 1 month.

▶ Redness of both eyes lasts more than 7 days.

▶ You have other questions or concerns.

Parent Care at Home If

▶ Pink/red eye is part of a cold.

▶ Pink/red eye is caused by mild irritant (such as soap, sunscreen, food, smoke, or chlorine).

Care Advice

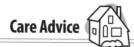

Treatment for Viral Eye Infections

❶ What You Should Know

- Some viruses cause watery eyes (viral conjunctivitis).

- It may be the first symptom of a cold.

- It isn't serious. You can treat this at home.

- Colds can cause a small amount of mucus in the corner of the eye.

- Here is some care advice that should help.

❷ Eyelid Rinse

- Cleanse eyelids with warm water and a clean cotton ball.

- Try to do this 3 times a day.

- This will usually keep a bacterial infection from occurring.

❸ Artificial Tears

- Artificial tears often make pink eyes feel better. No prescription is needed. They can be used at any age.

- Use 1 drop per eye 3 times a day as needed. Use them after cleansing the eyelids.

- Antibiotic and vasoconstrictor eyedrops do not help viral eye infections.

❹ Eyedrops: How to Use

- For a cooperative child, gently pull down on the lower lid. Put 1 drop inside the lower lid. Then ask your child to close the eye for 2 minutes. (**Reason:** So the medicine will get into the tissues.)

- For a child who won't open the eye, have them lie down. Put 1 drop over the inner corner of the eye. If your child opens the eye or blinks, the eyedrop will flow in. If they don't open the eye, the drop will slowly seep into it.

❺ Contact Lenses

- Children who wear contact lenses need to switch to glasses until the infection is gone.

- **Reason:** To prevent damage to the cornea.

❻ Return to School

- Pinkeye with watery discharge is harmless and mildly contagious.

- Children with pink eyes from a cold do not need to miss any school.

- Pinkeye is not a public health risk. Keeping these children home is overreacting. If asked, tell the school your child is on eyedrops (artificial tears).

❼ What to Expect

- Pinkeye with a cold usually lasts about 7 days.

- Sometimes, it turns into a bacterial eye infection. You can tell because the eyelids will become stuck together with pus. (See Chapter 9, Eye, Pus or Discharge.)

- Pinkeye from an irritant usually goes away within 2 hours after it's removed.

❽ Call Your Doctor If

- Your child gets pus in the eye.

- Redness of 1 eye lasts more than 1 day.

- Redness of both eyes lasts more than 1 week.

- You think your child needs to be seen.

- Your child becomes worse.

Treatment for Mild Eye Irritants

❶ What You Should Know About Pinkeye From Irritants

- Most eye irritants cause redness of the eyes.

- It will go away on its own.

- You can treat it at home.

❷ Face Wash

- Wash the face with mild soap and water.

- This will remove any irritants still on the face.

❸ Eyelid Rinse

- Rinse the eyelids with warm water for 5 minutes.

❹ Eyedrops

- Red eyes from irritants usually feel much better after being washed out.
- At any age, if eyes remain bloodshot, you can use artificial tears.
- If older than 6 years, switch to a long-acting vasoconstrictor eyedrop (such as Visine). No prescription is needed.
- **Dose:** Use 1 drop. May repeat once in 8 to 12 hours. Never use for more than 3 days.

❺ What to Expect

- After the irritant is removed, the eyes usually return to normal color.
- This may take 1 to 2 hours.

❻ Prevention

- Try to avoid future contact with the irritant.

❼ Call Your Doctor If

- Pus in the eye occurs.
- Eye becomes painful.
- Redness of 1 eye lasts more than 1 day.
- Redness of both eyes lasts more than 7 days.
- You think your child needs to be seen.
- Your child becomes worse.

Remember!
Contact your doctor if your child develops any of the **Call Your Doctor** symptoms.

CHAPTER 9

Eye, Pus or Discharge

Definition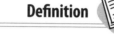

- ► Yellow or green discharge (pus) in the eye.
- ► The eyelids are stuck (matted) together with pus after sleep.
- ► After being wiped away, the pus comes back during the day.
- ► Often caused by a bacterial eye infection.

See Other Chapter If

- ► No pus in the eye. See Chapter 8, Eye, Red Without Pus.
- ► Main symptom is itchy eyes. See Chapter 10, Eye Allergy.

Causes of Eye With Pus

- ► **Bacterial conjunctivitis.** This is a bacterial infection of the eye. The main symptom is eyelids stuck together with pus after sleep. Can be present in 1 or both eyes. A few viruses can cause pus in the eyes, but most don't.

- ► **Viral conjunctivitis.** This is a viral infection of the eyes. Main symptom is pinkness of the white parts of the eyes. The eyes are also watery. Most often, there is no pus. Usually occurs on both sides.

- ► **Normal discharge.** A small amount of dried mucus only in the corner of the eye. It may not even be pus. A collection of mucus can be cream colored. Often due to an irritant that got in the eye from dirty hands. Needs no treatment except wiping it away with warm water.

- ► **Blocked tear duct.** Present in 10% of newborns. Main symptom is a constant watery eye. Tears fill the eye and run down the face. This happens even when not crying. The eye is not red and the eyelid is not swollen. The wet eye may get secondary infections. This will cause the eyelids to become matted with pus.

▸ **Foreign body (object) in the eye (serious).** Small particles such as sand, dirt, or saw-dust can be blown into the eyes. The grit often gets stuck under the upper eyelid. If not removed, the eye reacts by producing pus. The main clue is an eye infection that does not respond to antibiotic eyedrops. Older children report feeling something in the eye.

▸ **Eyelid cellulitis (serious).** This is a deep infection of the eyelid and tissues around it. The main symptom is a red, swollen, very tender eyelid. The eye can be swollen shut. Usually occurs only on one side. This can be a complication of bacterial conjunctivitis. The eye infection spreads inward. More commonly, this is caused by an ethmoid sinus infection. That type occurs without any pus in the eye.

Symptoms of Bacterial Eye Infection

▸ Yellow or green discharge or pus in the eye.

▸ Dried pus on the eyelids and eyelashes.

▸ The eyelashes are more likely to be stuck together after sleep.

▸ The whites of the eye may be red or pink.

▸ The eyelids are often puffy.

When to Call Your Doctor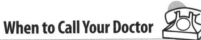

Call Your Doctor Now (Night or Day) If

▸ Eyelid is very red or very swollen.

▸ Vision is blurred.

▸ Eye pain present and more than mild.

▸ Fever higher than 104°F (40°C).

▸ **Age:** Younger than 12 weeks with fever. (**Caution:** Do *not* give your baby any fever medicine before being seen.)

▸ Your child looks or acts very sick.

▸ You think your child needs to be seen, and the problem is urgent.

Call Your Doctor Within 24 Hours If

▸ Pus in the eye but none of the symptoms above are present. (**Reason:** You may need antibiotic eyedrops to treat it.)

▸ Despite you using antibiotic eyedrops over 3 days, pus is still present.

Care Advice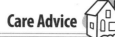

❶ What You Should Know About Bacterial Eye Infections

- Bacterial eye infections are common with colds.
- They respond to home treatment with antibiotic eyedrops, which need a prescription.
- They are not harmful to vision.
- Until you get some antibiotic eyedrops, here is some advice that should help.

❷ Remove Pus

- Remove all the dried and liquid pus from the eyelids. Use warm water and wet cotton balls to do this.
- Do this whenever pus is seen on the eyelids.
- Also, remove the pus before the antibiotic eyedrops are put in. (**Reason:** They will not work if you don't.)
- The pus can spread infection to others. So, dispose of cotton balls carefully.
- Wash your hands well after any contact with the eye or drainage.

❸ Antibiotic Eyedrops: How to Use

- For a cooperative child, gently pull down on the lower lid. Put 1 drop inside the lower lid. Then ask your child to close the eye for 2 minutes. (**Reason:** So the medicine will get into the tissues.)
- For a child who won't open his eye, have him lie down. Put 1 drop over the inner corner of the eye. If your child opens the eye or blinks, the eyedrop will flow in. If he doesn't open the eye, the drop will slowly seep into it.

❹ Contact Lenses

- Children who wear contact lenses need to switch to glasses until the infection is gone. (**Reason:** To prevent damage to the cornea.)
- Disinfect the lenses before wearing them again.
- Discard them if they are disposable.

❺ Return to School

- Your child can return to school when the pus is a small amount.
- Antibiotic eyedrops should be used for 24 hours before going back.

❻ What to Expect

- With treatment, the pus discharge should clear up in 3 days.
- Red eyes may last up to a week.

❼ Call Your Doctor If

- Eyelid gets red or swollen.
- You think your child needs to be seen.
- Your child becomes worse.

Remember!
Contact your doctor if your child develops any of the **Call Your Doctor** symptoms.

CHAPTER 10

Eye Allergy

Definition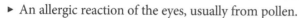

▸ An allergic reaction of the eyes, usually from pollen.

▸ The eyes are itchy and watery.

See Other Chapter If

▸ Runny, itchy nose and sneezing are also present. See Chapter 17, Nose Allergy (Hay Fever).

▸ Yellow or green pus in the eyes. See Chapter 9, Eye, Pus or Discharge.

▸ Doesn't look like an eye allergy. See Chapter 8, Eye, Red Without Pus.

Symptoms of Eye Allergies

▸ Itchy eyes (sometimes feels like burning or stinging).

▸ Increased tearing (watery eyes).

▸ Red or pink eyes.

▸ Mild swelling of the eyelids.

▸ No discharge or a sticky, stringy, mucus discharge.

▸ No pain or fever.

Triggers of Eye Allergies

▸ **Cause.** An allergic reaction of the eyes to an allergic substance. The medical name for this is *allergic conjunctivitis*. The allergic substance is called an *allergen*. Most allergens float in the air. That's how they get in the eyes. Here are the common ones.

   • **Pollens.** Trees, grass, weeds, and molds are the most common pollens. Tree pollens arrive in the spring. Grass pollens are present in the summer. Weed pollens come in the fall. Pollens cause seasonal eye allergies. You can't avoid pollens because they are in the air. Most eye allergies continue through pollen season. They can last 4 to 8 weeks.

- **Pets.** Allergens can also be from cats, dogs, horses, rabbits, and other animals. Pet allergens are in the air. They can also get in the eyes from the hands. Most people don't keep a pet that they are allergic to. They will only have sporadic allergic symptoms when they are exposed to the animal. These symptoms will usually last a few hours. If you own the pet, though, your child will have symptoms all the time.

- **House dust.** House dust contains many allergens. It always contains dust mites. If your humidity is high, it will contain mold. If people with a cat visit you, they will bring cat dander with them. House dust causes year-round, daily symptoms. The medical name for this is *perennial eye allergies.*

When to Call Your Doctor

Call Your Doctor Within 24 Hours If

▶ You think your child needs to be seen.

▶ Sacs of clear fluid (blisters) on whites of the eyes.

▶ Eyelids are swollen shut (or almost shut).

▶ Discharge on eyelids does not go away with allergy medicines.

Call Your Doctor During Weekday Office Hours If

▶ Eyes are very itchy after taking allergy medicines for more than 2 days.

▶ Diagnosis of eye allergy never made by a doctor.

▶ You have other questions or concerns.

Parent Care at Home If

▶ Mild eye allergy.

Care Advice

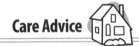

❶ What You Should Know About Eye Allergies

■ An eye allergy is most often caused by pollen that gets in the eye.

■ The eyes can itch, burn, or sting.

■ All of these symptoms can go away with allergy eyedrops.

■ Eye allergies are common. They occur in 10% of children.

■ Here is some care advice that should help.

❷ Wash Allergens Off the Face

- Use a wet washcloth to clean off the eyelids and face.
- Rinse the eyes with a small amount of warm water. Tears will do the rest.
- Then put a cold, wet washcloth on the itchy eye.
- Prevention: Wash your child's hair every night because it collects lots of pollen.

❸ Oral Allergy Medicines

- If the nose is also itchy and runny, your child probably has hay fever. Hay fever is allergic symptoms of both the nose and eyes.
- Give your child an allergy medicine by mouth. This should get rid of the nose and eye symptoms. Sometimes, then eyedrops will not be needed.
- Long-acting allergy medicines (such as Zyrtec) are best. No prescription is needed. This kind of medicine has 2 advantages over Benadryl. It causes less sedation and lasts up to 24 hours. Age limit: 2 years or older.
- Give allergy medicine every day. Do this until pollen season is over (about 2 months for each pollen).

❹ Antihistamine Eyedrops (Ketotifen) for Pollen Allergies: First Choice

- Usually, an oral allergy medicine will control allergic symptoms of the eye.
- If the eyes remain itchy and poorly controlled, purchase some Ketotifen antihistamine eyedrops. Ask your pharmacist to suggest a brand (such as Zaditor). No prescription is needed.
- **Age:** Approved for 3 years and older.
- **Dose:** 1 drop every 12 hours in both eyes.
- For severe allergies, use of ketotifen eyedrops every day will help the most. Use these eyedrops until pollen season is over.

❺ Older Antihistamine/Vasoconstrictor Eyedrops: Second Choice

- Often, the eyes will feel much better after the allergic substance is washed out. Also, putting a cold, wet washcloth on them usually makes them feel better.
- If not, this type of eyedrop can be used for added relief. Ask your pharmacist to suggest a brand (such as Visine-A; the *A* stands for antihistamine). No prescription is needed.
- Avoid vasoconstrictor eyedrops without an allergy medicine in them. These are the eyedrops without an *A* in the name, such as plain Visine. (**Reason:** They treat only redness, not the cause.)

- **Dose:** 1 drop every 8 hours as needed.
- Do not use for more than 5 days. (**Reason:** Will cause red eyes from rebound effect.)
- Downside: Doesn't work as well as ketotifen eyedrops.

❻ Eyedrops: How to Use

- For a cooperative child, gently pull down on the lower lid. Put 1 drop inside the lower lid. Then ask your child to close the eye for 2 minutes. (**Reason:** So the medicine will get into the tissues.)
- For a child who won't open her eye, have her lie down. Put 1 drop over the inner corner of the eye. If your child opens the eye or blinks, the eyedrop will flow in. If she doesn't open the eye, the drop will slowly seep into it.

❼ Contact Lenses

- Children who wear contact lenses may need to switch to glasses for a while.
- This will help the eye heal faster.

❽ What to Expect

- If you know the cause of the allergic symptoms, try to avoid it. This is the case with animal allergies. Symptoms will not come back if there is no contact.
- You can't avoid pollens because they are in the air. Most eye allergies continue through pollen season. They can last 4 to 8 weeks.

❾ Call Your Doctor If

- Itchy eyes aren't better in 2 days with allergy treatment.
- You think your child needs to be seen.
- Your child becomes worse.

Remember!
Contact your doctor if your child develops any of
the **Call Your Doctor** symptoms.

PART 4

Ear Symptoms

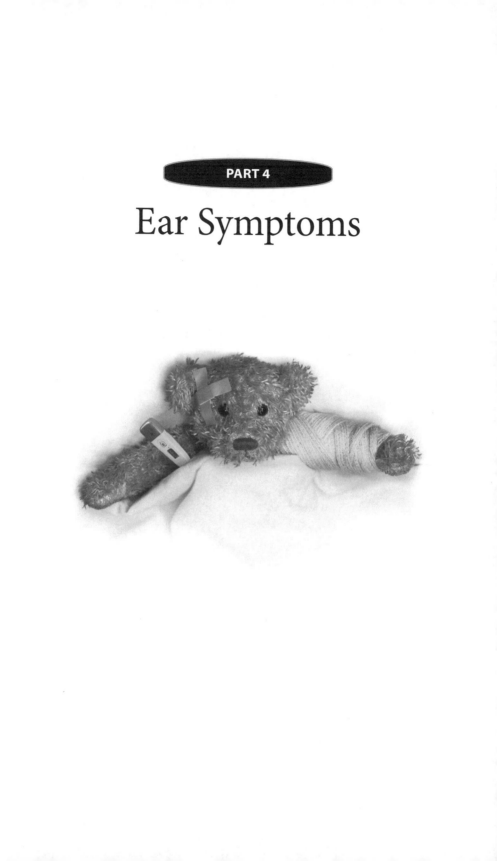

CHAPTER 11

Earache

Definition

▶ Pain in or around the ear.

▶ The older child reports ear pain.

▶ Younger child acts like he did with last ear infection or cries a lot.

▶ Earache not caused by an ear injury.

Causes of Earaches

▶ **Ear infection.** An infection of the middle ear (space behind the eardrum) is the most common cause. Ear infections can be caused by viruses or bacteria. Usually, a doctor can tell the difference by looking at the eardrum.

▶ **Swimmer's ear.** An infection or irritation of the skin that lines the ear canal. Main symptom is itchy ear canal. If the canal becomes infected, it also becomes painful. Mainly occurs in swimmers and in the summertime.

▶ **Ear canal injury.** A cotton swab or fingernail can cause a scrape in the canal.

▶ **Ear canal abscess.** An infection of a hair follicle in the ear canal can be very painful. It looks like a small red bump. Sometimes, it turns into a pimple and needs to be drained.

▶ **Earwax.** A big piece of hard earwax can cause mild ear pain. If the wax has been pushed in by cotton swabs, the ear canal can become blocked. This pain will be worse.

▶ **Ear canal foreign body (object).** Young children may put small objects in their ear canal. It will cause pain if object is sharp or pushed in very far.

▶ **Airplane ear.** If the ear tube is blocked, sudden increases in air pressure can cause the eardrum to stretch. The main symptom is severe ear pain. It usually starts when coming down for a landing. It can also occur during mountain driving.

▶ **Pierced ear infections.** These infections are common. If not treated early, they can become very painful.

▸ **Referred pain.** Ear pain can also be referred (coming) from diseases not in the ear. Tonsil infections are a common example. Tooth decay in a back molar can feel like ear pain. Mumps can be reported as ear pain. (**Reason:** The mumps parotid gland is in front of the ear.) Jaw pain (TMJ [temporomandibular joint] syndrome) can masquerade as ear pain.

Ear Infections: Most Common Cause

▸ **Definition.** An infection of the middle ear (space behind the eardrum). Viral ear infections are more common than bacterial ones.

▸ **Symptoms.** The main symptom is an earache. Younger children will cry, act fussy, or have trouble sleeping because of pain. About 50% of children with an ear infection will have a fever.

▸ **Diagnosis.** A doctor can diagnose a bacterial ear infection by looking at the eardrum. It will bulge and have pus behind it. For viral ear infections, the eardrum will be red but not bulging.

▸ **Age range.** Ear infections peak at age 6 months to 2 years. They are a common problem until age 8. The onset of ear infections is often on day 3 of a cold.

▸ **Frequency.** Ninety percent of children have at least 1 ear infection. Frequent ear infections occur in 20% of children. Ear infections are the most common bacterial infection of young children.

▸ **Complication of bacterial ear infections.** In 5% to 10% of children, the eardrum will develop a small tear. This is from pressure in the middle ear. The ear then drains cloudy fluid or pus. This small hole most often heals in 2 or 3 days.

▸ **Treatment.** Bacterial ear infections need an oral antibiotic. Viral ear infections get better on their own. Children need pain medicine and supportive care.

When to Call Your Doctor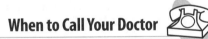

Call 911 Now (Your Child May Need an Ambulance) If

▸ Not moving or too weak to stand.

▸ You think your child has a life-threatening emergency.

Go to ER Now

▸ Not alert when awake (out of it).

Call Your Doctor Now (Night or Day) If

▶ Severe earache has not improved 2 hours after taking ibuprofen.

▶ Pink or red swelling behind the ear.

▶ Outer ear is red, swollen, and painful.

▶ Stiff neck and can't touch chin to chest.

▶ Walking is not steady.

▶ Pointed object was put into the ear canal (such as a pencil, stick, or wire).

▶ Weak immune system (such as sickle cell disease, HIV, cancer, organ transplant, or taking oral steroids).

▶ Fever higher than 104°F (40°C).

▶ Your child looks or acts very sick.

▶ You think your child needs to be seen, and the problem is urgent.

Call Your Doctor Within 24 Hours If

▶ Earache but none of the symptoms above. (**Reason:** Could be an ear infection.)

▶ Pus or cloudy discharge from ear canal.

Care Advice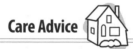

❶ What You Should Know About Earaches

▪ Your child may have an ear infection. The only way to be sure is to look at the eardrum.

▪ It is safe to wait until your doctor's office is open to call. It is not harmful to wait if the pain starts at night.

▪ Ear pain can usually be controlled with pain medicine.

▪ Many earaches are caused by a virus and don't need an antibiotic.

▪ Here is some care advice that should help until you talk with your doctor.

❷ Pain Medicine

▪ To help with the pain, give an acetaminophen product (such as Tylenol).

▪ Another choice is an ibuprofen product (such as Advil).

▪ Use as needed.

❸ Cold Pack for Pain

- Put a cold, wet washcloth on the outer ear for 20 minutes. This should help ease pain until the pain medicine starts to work.

- **Note:** Some children prefer heat for 20 minutes.

- **Caution:** Heat or cold kept on too long could cause a burn or frostbite.

❹ Ear Infection Discharge

- If pus is draining from the ear, the eardrum probably has a small tear. Usually, this is from an ear infection. Discharge can also occur if your child has ear tubes.

- The pus may be blood tinged.

- Most often, this heals well after the ear infection is treated.

- Wipe the discharge away as you see it.

- Do not plug the ear canal with cotton. (**Reason:** Retained pus can infect lining of the ear canal.)

❺ Fever Medicine

- For fevers above 102°F (39°C), give an acetaminophen product (such as Tylenol).

- Another choice is an ibuprofen product (such as Advil).

- **Note:** Fevers below 102°F (39°C) are important for fighting infections.

- **For all fevers:** Keep your child well hydrated. Give lots of cold fluids.

❻ Return to School

- Ear infections cannot be spread to others.

- Can return to school or child care when the fever is gone.

❼ Call Your Doctor If

- Pain becomes severe.

- You think your child needs to be seen.

- Your child becomes worse.

Remember!
Contact your doctor if your child develops any of
the **Call Your Doctor** symptoms.

CHAPTER 12

Ear, Pulling At or Rubbing

Definition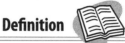

▶ A child who pulls, tugs, pokes, rubs, or itches the ear.

▶ Most ear pulling or touching is normal behavior (age 4–12 months).

▶ No crying or report of ear pain.

See Other Chapter If

▶ Child is crying, and ear pulling is minor or normal. See Chapter 7, Crying Child.

▶ Child reports ear pain. See Chapter 11, Earache.

▶ Earwax buildup is the problem. See Chapter 14, Earwax Buildup.

Causes of Ear Pulling

▶ **Habit.** Main cause in infants. Normal touching and pulling with discovery of ears. This is usually not seen before 4 months of age or continued after 12 months.

▶ **Earwax.** The main cause in older children is a piece of earwax. This earwax build-up is usually caused by putting cotton swabs in the ear canal. Until the teen years, cotton swabs are wider than the ear canal. Therefore, they push earwax back in.

▶ **Soap.** Another cause of an itchy ear canal is soap or other irritants. Soap or shampoo can get trapped in the ear canal after showers.

▶ **Ear infection.** Children with ear infections act sick. They present with an earache or unexplained crying.

▶ **Note:** Rubbing the ear is common in children younger than 2 or 3 years. Simple ear pulling without other symptoms such as fever or crying is harmless. These children rarely have an ear infection.

When to Call Your Doctor

Call Your Doctor Now (Night or Day) If

▸ Fever above 104°F (40°C).

▸ **Age:** Younger than 12 weeks with fever. (**Caution:** Do *not* give your baby any fever medicine before being seen.)

▸ Your child looks or acts very sick.

▸ You think your child needs to be seen, and the problem is urgent.

Call Your Doctor Within 24 Hours If

▸ Seems to be in pain (or is crying).

▸ Starts to wake up from sleep.

▸ Fever or symptoms of a cold are present.

▸ Drainage from the ear canal.

▸ Frequent digging inside 1 ear canal.

▸ You think your child needs to be seen, but the problem is not urgent.

Call Your Doctor During Weekday Office Hours If

▸ Pulling at or rubbing the ear lasts more than 3 days.

▸ Itching lasts more than 1 week.

▸ You have other questions or concerns.

Parent Care at Home If

▸ Normal ear touching or pulling.

▸ Itchy ear canal.

Care Advice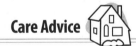

❶ What You Should Know About Ear Rubbing

▪ Most infants have discovered their ears and are playing with them.

▪ Some have an itchy ear canal.

- Earwax buildup is the most common cause. Most wax problems are caused by putting cotton swabs in the ear canal.

- Ear pulling can start when your child has a cold. It can be caused by fluid in the middle ear. Less often, it's caused by an ear infection. If this is the case, your child will develop other symptoms. Look for fever or increased crying.

- Ear pulling without other symptoms is not a sign of an ear infection.

- Here is some care advice that should help.

❷ Habit Type of Ear Rubbing

- If touching the ear is a new habit, ignore it.

- This helps prevent your child from doing it for attention.

❸ Cotton Swabs: Do Not Use

- Cotton swabs can push earwax back and cause a plug.

- Earwax has a purpose. It protects lining of the ear canal.

- Earwax comes out on its own.

- Cotton swabs should never be used before the teen years. (**Reason:** They are wider than the ear canal.)

❹ Keep Soap Out of the Ears

- Keep soap and shampoo out of the ear canal to prevent itchiness.

❺ White Vinegar Eardrops

- For an itchy ear canal, you can use half-strength white vinegar. Make this by mixing the vinegar with equal parts warm water.

- Place 2 drops in each ear canal once daily.

- Do this for 3 days.

- **Reason:** Restores normal acid pH.

- **Caution:** Do not use eardrops if your child has ear drainage or ear tubes. Also, do not use them if your child has a hole in the eardrum.

❻ What to Expect

- With this treatment, most itching is gone in 2 or 3 days.

❼ Call Your Doctor If

- Rubbing of ear lasts more than 3 days.
- Itching of ear lasts more than 1 week.
- You think your child needs to be seen.
- Your child becomes worse.

Remember!
Contact your doctor if your child develops any of the **Call Your Doctor** symptoms.

CHAPTER 13

Ear Infection

Definition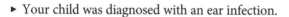

- ▸ Your child was diagnosed with an ear infection.
- ▸ Your child's ears were recently looked at by a doctor.
- ▸ You are worried that the fever or ear pain is not getting better fast enough.
- ▸ Your child is still taking an antibiotic for the ear infection.

Symptoms of Ear Infections

- ▸ The main symptom is an earache.
- ▸ Younger children will cry, act fussy, or have trouble sleeping because of pain.
- ▸ About 50% of children with an ear infection will have a fever.
- ▸ **Complication:** In 5% to 10% of children, the eardrum will develop a small tear. This is from pressure in the middle ear. The ear then drains cloudy fluid or pus. This small hole most often heals in 2 or 3 days.

Cause of Ear Infections

- ▸ A bacterial infection of the middle ear (space behind the eardrum).
- ▸ Blocked eustachian tube, usually as part of a common cold. The eustachian tube joins the middle ear to the back of the throat.
- ▸ Blockage results in middle ear fluid (called *viral otitis*).
- ▸ If the fluid becomes infected (*bacterial otitis*), it turns to pus. This causes the eardrum to bulge out and can cause a lot of pain.
- ▸ Ear infections peak at age 6 months to 2 years. They are a common problem until age 8.
- ▸ The onset of ear infections is often on day 3 of a cold.
- ▸ How often do children get ear infections? Approximately 90% of children have at least 1 ear infection during the early years. Frequent ear infections occur in 20% of children. Ear infections are the most common bacterial infection in young children.

When to Call Your Doctor

Call 911 Now (Your Child May Need an Ambulance) If

▶ Not moving or too weak to stand.

▶ You think your child has a life-threatening emergency.

Call Your Doctor Now (Night or Day) If

▶ Stiff neck (can't touch the chin to chest).

▶ Walking is not steady.

▶ Fever above 104°F (40°C).

▶ Ear pain is severe and doesn't improve 2 hours after taking ibuprofen.

▶ Crying is inconsolable and doesn't improve 2 hours after taking ibuprofen.

▶ Pink or red swelling behind the ear.

▶ Crooked smile (weakness of 1 side of the face).

▶ New vomiting.

▶ Your child looks or acts very sick.

▶ You think your child needs to be seen, and the problem is urgent.

Call Your Doctor Within 24 Hours If

▶ Taking antibiotic more than 48 hours and fever still present or comes back.

▶ Taking antibiotic more than 3 days and ear pain is not better.

▶ Taking antibiotic over 3 days and ear discharge still present or comes back.

▶ You think your child needs to be seen, but the problem is not urgent.

Call Your Doctor During Weekday Office Hours If

▶ You have other questions or concerns.

Parent Care at Home If

▶ Ear infection on antibiotic with no complications.

▶ Normal hearing loss with an ear infection.

▶ Prevention of ear infections.

▶ Ear (ventilation) tube surgery questions.

Care Advice

Treatment for an Ear Infection

❶ What You Should Know About Ear Infections

- Ear infections are very common in young children.

- Most ear infections are not cured after the first dose of antibiotic.

- Often, children don't get better during the first day.

- Most children get better slowly over 2 to 3 days.

- **Note:** For mild ear infections in older children, antibiotics may not be needed. This is an option if the child is older than 2 years and infection looks viral, and if the child can report whether the symptoms are getting better or worse.

- Here is some care advice that should help.

❷ Keep Giving the Antibiotic

- The antibiotic will kill bacteria that are causing the ear infection.

- Try not to forget any doses.

- Give the antibiotic until it is gone. (**Reason:** To stop ear infection from flaring up again.)

❸ Fever Medicine

- For fevers above 102°F (39°C), give an acetaminophen product (such as Tylenol).

- Another choice is an ibuprofen product (such as Advil).

- **Note:** Fevers below 102°F (39°C) are important for fighting infections.

- **For all fevers:** Keep your child well hydrated. Give lots of cold fluids.

❹ Pain Medicine

- To help with pain, give an acetaminophen product (such as Tylenol).

- Another choice is an ibuprofen product (such as Advil).

- Use as needed.

❺ Cold Pack for Pain

- Put a cold, wet washcloth on the outer ear for 20 minutes. This should help ease pain until the pain medicine starts to work.

- **Note:** Some children prefer heat for 20 minutes.

- **Caution:** Heat or cold kept on too long could cause a burn or frostbite.

❻ Limits on Activity

- Your child can go outside and does not need to cover her ears.

- Swimming is fine as long as no drainage is coming from the ear. Also, do not swim if there is a tear in the eardrum.

- Air travel
  - Children with ear infections can travel safely by aircraft if they are taking antibiotics. For most, flying will not make their ear pain worse.
  - Give your child a dose of ibuprofen 1 hour before takeoff. This will help with any pain she might have. Also, during descent (coming down for landing) have your child swallow fluids. Sucking on a pacifier may help as well. Children older than 6 years can chew gum.

❼ Return to School

- Your child can go back to school or child care when the fever is gone.

- Your child feels well enough to join in normal activities.

- Ear infections cannot be spread to others.

❽ What to Expect

- Once on antibiotics, your child will get better in 2 or 3 days.

- Make sure you give your child the antibiotic as directed.

- The fever should be gone within 2 days (48 hours).

- The ear pain should be better within 2 days. It should be gone within 3 days (72 hours).

❾ Ear Infection Discharge

- If pus is draining from the ear, the eardrum probably has a small tear. This can be normal with an ear infection. Discharge can also occur if your child has ear tubes.

- The pus may be blood tinged.

- Most often, this heals well after the ear infection is treated.

- Wipe the discharge away as you see it.

- Do not plug the ear canal with cotton. (**Reason:** Retained pus can infect lining of the ear canal.)

❿ Call Your Doctor If

- Fever lasts more than 2 days on antibiotics.

- Ear pain becomes severe or crying becomes nonstop.

- Ear pain lasts more than 3 days on antibiotics.
- Ear discharge is not better after 3 days on antibiotics.
- You think your child needs to be seen.
- Your child becomes worse.

Treatment for Hearing Loss With an Ear Infection

❶ Brief Hearing Loss

- During an ear infection, fluid builds up in the middle ear space.
- Fluid can cause a mild hearing loss for a short time.
- It will slowly get better and go away with an antibiotic.
- Fluid will no longer be infected but, sometimes, may take weeks to go away. In 90% of children, it clears up by itself over 1 to 2 months.
- Permanent harm in hearing is very rare.

❷ Talking With Your Child

- Get close to your child and maintain eye contact.
- Speak in a louder voice than you usually use.
- Decrease any background noise from the radio or TV while talking with your child.

❸ Call Your Doctor If

- Hearing loss doesn't improve after the antibiotic is done.

Prevention of Recurrent Ear Infections

❶ What You Should Know

- Some children have ear infections that keep coming back.
- If your child experiences recurrent ear infections, here are some ways to prevent future ones.

❷ Avoid Tobacco Smoke

- Contact with tobacco smoke can lead to ear infections.
- It also makes them harder to treat.
- No one should smoke around your child. This includes in your home, your car, or at child care.

❸ Avoid Colds

- Most ear infections start with a cold. During the first year of life, try to minimize contact with other sick children.

- Try to delay using a large child care center during the first year. Instead, try using a sitter in your home. Another option might be a small home-based child care.

❹ Breastfeed

- Breastfeed your baby during the first 6 to 12 months of life.

- Antibodies in breast milk lower the rate of ear infections.

- If you breastfeed, continue it.

- If you do not, consider it with your next child.

❺ Do Not Prop the Bottle

- During feedings, hold your baby with the head higher than the stomach.

- Feeding while lying down flat can lead to ear infections. It causes formula to flow back into the middle ear.

- Having babies hold their own bottle also causes milk to drain into the middle ear.

❻ Get All Suggested Vaccines

- Vaccines protect your child from serious infections.

- The pneumococcal and flu shots also help prevent some ear infections.

❼ Control Allergies

- Allergies may lead to some ear infections.

- If your baby has a constant runny or blocked nose, suspect an allergy.

- If your child has other allergies like eczema, ask your child's doctor about this. The doctor can check for a milk or soy protein allergy.

❽ Check Any Snoring

- Large adenoids can cause snoring or mouth breathing. Suspect this if your toddler snores every night or breathes through her mouth.

- Large adenoids can contribute to ear infections.

- Talk with your child's doctor about this.

Ear Tube Surgery Questions

❶ Ear Tubes

- Ear tubes are tiny plastic tubes put through the eardrum. They are placed by an ear, nose, and throat doctor.

- The tubes allow fluid to drain out of the middle ear space. They also allow air to reenter the space.

- This lowers the risk of repeated ear infections and returns hearing to normal.

❷ Ear Tubes: When Are They Needed?

- Fluid has been present in the middle ear nonstop for more than 4 months. Both ears have fluid.

- Also, the fluid has caused a hearing loss greater than 20 decibels.

- Hearing should be tested first. Some children have nearly normal hearing and tubes are not needed.

- Ear infections that do not clear up after trying many antibiotics may need tubes.

- Prevention should be tried before turning to surgery.

- Talk with your child's doctor about when ear tubes are needed.

❸ What to Expect

- In most cases, the tubes come out after about a year. They fall out of the ear on their own. This happens with the normal movement of earwax.

- If the tubes stay in more than 2 years, talk with your child's doctor. The surgeon may need to take them out.

❹ Risks of Ear Tubes

- After the tubes come out, they may leave scars on the eardrum. They may also leave a small hole that doesn't heal. Both of these problems can cause a small hearing loss.

- Because of these possible complications, there is a small risk with ear tubes. There is also a small risk when giving anesthesia to young children.

- Therefore, doctors suggest ear tubes only for children who really need them.

Remember!
Contact your doctor if your child develops any of the **Call Your Doctor** symptoms.

CHAPTER 14

Earwax Buildup

Definition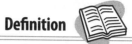

- ▶ Symptoms and causes of earwax (cerumen) buildup or blockage.
- ▶ Questions about earwax removal.

See Other Chapter If

- ▶ Pain in or around ear is main symptom. See Chapter 11, Earache.

Symptoms of Earwax Buildup

- ▶ Too much earwax can cause rubbing of the ear or poking in the canal.
- ▶ A piece of ear wax can become dry and hard in the ear canal. This creates a feeling that an object is in the ear.
- ▶ Complete blockage (plugging) of the ear canal by wax causes more symptoms. These include decreased or muffled hearing.
- ▶ A large piece of earwax may be seen inside the ear canal.

Causes of Earwax Buildup

- ▶ **Cotton swabs.** Earwax buildup is usually from using cotton swabs. They push wax back in and pack it down.
- ▶ **Fingers.** A few children (perhaps 5%) normally produce more wax than others. It will usually come out if it's not pushed back by fingers.
- ▶ **Earplugs.** Wearing earplugs of any type can also push wax back.

Earwax Is Normal

- ▶ Everyone has earwax. Earwax is normal and healthy. It is not dirty or a sign of poor hygiene.
- ▶ Earwax is also called *cerumen.*
- ▶ Earwax is made by special glands in the outer third part of the ear canal.
- ▶ Earwax has a purpose. It protects skin lining the ear canal. It is a natural waterproofing agent.

▶ Earwax also has germ-killing properties.

▶ New earwax is soft and a golden-yellow color.

▶ Older earwax becomes dryer and turns to a brown or black color.

Ear Canals Are Self-cleaning

▶ Ear canals are designed to clean themselves.

▶ Ear canal skin slowly moves out of the ear canal. It carries earwax along with it. The wax dries up and becomes flaky. It falls out of the ear on its own.

▶ Some people produce much more earwax than others. For such people, periodic ear cleaning may be needed.

▶ Earwax needs to be removed from inside the ear only if it causes symptoms. Examples of symptoms are decreased hearing, discomfort, fullness, or blockage.

Problems From Using Cotton Swabs

▶ A cotton swab pushes wax back in. Then earwax builds up and causes symptoms.

▶ Ear canal blockage.

▶ Decreased or muffled hearing.

▶ Trapped water behind the wax (can lead to swimmer's ear).

▶ Itchy or painful canals, especially in teens who frequently use cotton swabs. A dry ear canal is always itchy.

▶ Sometimes, there can be bleeding or damage to the eardrum.

▶ Cotton swabs cause over 10,000 ear injuries each year in the United States. More than 2,000 are punctured eardrums. Never allow young children to play with cotton swabs.

Prevention of Blocked Ear Canals

▶ Never put cotton swabs (cotton buds or Q-tips) into the ear canal.

▶ Cotton swabs just push earwax deeper into the ear canal. (**Reason:** Cotton swabs are usually wider than a child's ear canal.)

▶ Earwax doesn't need any help getting out. You can't hurry the process.

▶ Never try to dig out pieces of earwax with toothpicks, matchsticks, or other devices. Usually, doing this just pushes wax back in.

▶ These objects can also scratch the ear canal and cause an infection.

► If all earwax is removed (as with cotton swabs), the ear canals become itchy. They also become more prone to swimmer's ear. This can occur in teens when cotton swabs are smaller than the ear canal.

► Limit the use of earplugs.

When to Call Your Doctor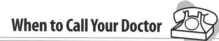

Call Your Doctor Now (Night or Day) If

► Ear pain or bleeding after an object (such as a cotton swab) was inserted into the ear canal.

► Ear pain after ear canal flushing to remove wax and it's severe.

► Walking is very unsteady.

► Your child looks or acts very sick.

► You think your child needs to be seen, and the problem is urgent.

Call Your Doctor Within 24 Hours If

► Ear pain after ear canal flushing lasts more than 1 hour.

► Pus (yellow or green discharge) from the ear canal.

► You think your child needs to be seen, but the problem is not urgent.

Call Your Doctor During Weekday Office Hours If

► History of ear drum perforation, tubes, or ear surgery. (**Reason:** Don't remove wax at home.)

► Complete hearing loss in either ear.

► **Age:** Younger than 6 years with earwax problems.

► Earwax problems not better after using this chapter's Care Advice.

► You don't want to try to remove earwax at home.

► You have other questions or concerns.

Parent Care at Home If

► You have questions about earwax removal.

Care Advice

❶ What You Should Know About Earwax Buildup

- Earwax is good.

- In general, leave earwax alone.

- It will come out on its own.

- If you see some wax right at the opening, you can remove it. Use something that won't push it back in.

❷ Reasons to Flush Out the Ear Canal

- Earwax is completely blocking an ear canal and can't hear on that side.

- If hearing seems normal on that side, blockage is only partial. You can leave it alone.

❸ 6 Years and Older: Ear Canal Flushing With Water

- For babies or children younger than 6, use only if advised by your child's doctor.

- Buy a soft rubber ear syringe or bulb from the pharmacy. No prescription is needed.

- Have your child lean over the sink. (**Reason:** To catch the water.)

- Use lukewarm water (body temperature). (**Reason:** To prevent dizziness.)

- Gently squirt the water into the ear canal. Then tilt your child's head and let the water run out. You may need to do this several (3–4) times.

- If the earwax does not seem to be coming out, tilt the head. Then, flush the earwax with the head tilted. Keep the ear with wax in it facing downward. Gravity will help the water wash it out (the waterfall effect).

- End point: Flush until the water that comes out is clear of wax. Also, the ear canal should be open when you look in with a light.

- Afterward, dry the ear thoroughly. You can do this by putting a drop of rubbing alcohol in the ear canal. Or you can set a hair dryer on low. Hold it a foot away from the ear for about 10 seconds.

❹ Caution: Ear Canal Flushing

■ Do not perform flushing if your child has a hole in the eardrum or ear tubes.

■ Stop flushing if it causes pain or dizziness.

■ Do not use a water jet tooth cleaner (such as a WaterPik) for ear flushing. (**Reason:** Force of the jet can cause pain.)

❺ Eardrops: Use for 4 Days to Soften the Earwax

■ If the earwax is hard, soften it before flushing the ear canal. Use eardrops to break up the earwax.

■ **Homemade eardrops:** Hydrogen peroxide and water solution. Mix equal parts of each. Or ask your doctor for what they prefer.

■ **Drugstore option:** Earwax removal eardrops (such as Debrox). No prescription is needed.

■ Use 5 drops in affected ear 2 times daily for 4 days.

❻ How to Put in Eardrops

■ Have your child lie on his side with the blocked ear upward.

■ Place 5 drops into ear canal.

■ Keep drops in ear for 10 minutes by continuing to lie down.

■ Then, roll over and lie with the blocked side down. Let the eardrops run out on some tissue.

■ Use twice daily for up to 4 days.

■ Follow up with flushing to get everything out.

❼ Cautions for Eardrops

■ Do not use eardrops if your child has a hole in the eardrum. Also, do not use them for children with ear tubes.

■ Stop using eardrops if pain occurs.

❽ Earwax Removal Before 6 Years of Age

■ Earwax removal in this age group can be hard.

■ Removal may not be needed. The earwax should come out on its own. Don't use cotton swabs.

■ Do not use eardrops or ear flushes unless it is advised by your child's doctor. This can also be done in your doctor's office.

❾ Call Your Doctor If

- Flushing out the ear canal doesn't return hearing to normal.

- Earache occurs.

- You think your child needs to be seen.

- Your child becomes worse.

Remember!
Contact your doctor if your child develops any of the **Call Your Doctor** symptoms.

PART 5

Nose Symptoms

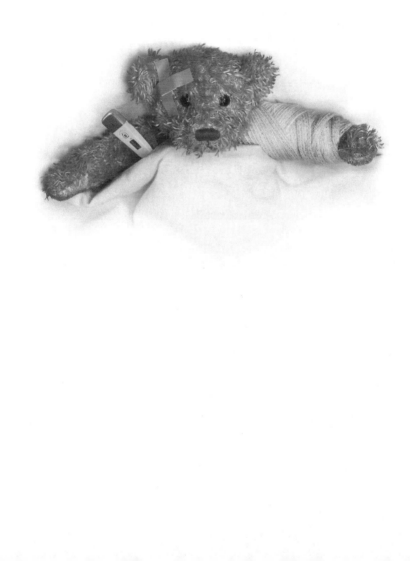

CHAPTER 15

Colds

Definition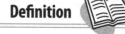

- ▶ Runny nose and sore throat caused by a virus.
- ▶ You think your child has a cold. (**Reason:** Other family members, friends or classmates have same symptoms.)
- ▶ Also called an *upper respiratory tract infection.*

See Other Chapter If

- ▶ Runny nose caused by allergies. See Chapter 17, Nose Allergy (Hay Fever).
- ▶ Cough is the main symptom. See Chapter 26, Cough.
- ▶ **Age:** Older than 5 years and pain around the eye or over the cheekbone. See Chapter 16, Sinus Pain or Congestion.

Symptoms of a Cold

- ▶ Runny or stuffy nose.
- ▶ Nasal discharge starts clear but changes to gray. It can also be yellow or green.
- ▶ Most children have a fever at the start.
- ▶ A sore throat can be the first sign.
- ▶ At times, the child may also have a cough and hoarse voice. Sometimes, watery eyes and swollen lymph nodes in the neck also occur.

Cause of Colds

- ▶ Colds are caused by many respiratory viruses. Healthy children get about 6 colds a year.
- ▶ Influenza virus causes a bad cold with more fever and muscle aches.
- ▶ Colds are not serious. With a cold, about 5% to 10% of children develop a complication. Most often, this is an ear or sinus infection. These are caused by a bacteria.

Colds: Normal Viral Symptoms

▸ Colds can cause a runny nose, sore throat, hoarse voice, a cough, or croup. They can also cause stuffiness of the nose, sinus, or ear. Red, watery eyes can also occur. Colds are the most common reason for calls to the doctor. This is because of all the symptoms that occur with colds.

▸ Cold symptoms are also the number one reason for office and ER visits. Advice in this chapter can help you avoid some trips to the doctor. Cold symptoms listed below are normal. These children don't need to be seen by a doctor.

• Fever up to 3 days (unless it goes above 104°F or 40°C).

• Sore throat up to 5 days (with other cold symptoms).

• Nasal discharge and congestion up to 2 weeks.

• Cough up to 3 weeks.

Colds: Symptoms of Secondary Bacterial Infections (Complications)

▸ Using advice in this chapter, you can decide if your child has developed a complication. This happens in about 5% to 10% of children who have a cold. Many will have an ear or a sinus infection. Look for the following symptoms:

• Earache or ear discharge.

• Sinus pain not relieved by nasal washes.

• Lots of pus in the eyes (eyelids stuck together after naps).

• Trouble breathing or rapid breathing (could have pneumonia).

• Fever lasts more than 3 days.

• Fever goes away for 24 hours and then returns.

• Sore throat lasts more than 5 days (may have strep throat infection [Chapter 20]).

• Nasal discharge lasts more than 2 weeks.

• Cough lasts more than 3 weeks.

Trouble Breathing: How to Tell

▸ Trouble breathing is a reason to see the doctor right away. *Respiratory distress* is the medical name for trouble breathing. Here are some symptoms of concern.

• Struggling for each breath or shortness of breath.

• Tight breathing where your child can barely speak or cry.

• Ribs are pulling in with each breath (called *retractions*).

- Breathing has become noisy (such as wheezes).
- Breathing is much faster than normal.
- Lips or face turn a blue color.

When to Call Your Doctor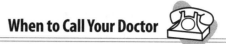

Call 911 Now (Your Child May Need an Ambulance) If

▸ Severe trouble breathing (struggling for each breath, can barely speak or cry).

▸ You think your child has a life-threatening emergency.

Go to ER Now If

▸ Ribs are pulling in with each breath (called *retractions*).

Call Your Doctor Now (Night or Day) If

▸ Not alert when awake (out of it).

▸ Trouble breathing, but not severe.

▸ Wheezing (purring or whistling sound) occurs.

▸ Breathing is much faster than normal.

▸ Trouble swallowing and new-onset drooling.

▸ High-risk child (such as with chronic lung disease).

▸ Weak immune system (such as sickle cell disease, HIV, cancer, organ transplant, or taking oral steroids).

▸ Fever above 104°F (40°C).

▸ **Age:** Younger than 12 weeks with fever. (**Caution:** Do *not* give your baby any fever medicine before being seen.)

▸ Your child looks or acts very sick.

▸ You think your child needs to be seen, and the problem is urgent.

Call Your Doctor Within 24 Hours If

▸ **Age:** Younger than 6 months.

▸ Earache or ear discharge.

▸ Yellow or green eye discharge.

▸ Sinus pain around cheekbone or eyes (not just congestion).

▸ Fever lasts more than 3 days.

▸ Fever returns after being gone for more than 24 hours.

▸ You think your child needs to be seen, but the problem is not urgent.

Call Your Doctor During Weekday Office Hours If

▸ Blocked nose and wakes up from sleep.

▸ Yellow scabs around nasal openings. (Use an antibiotic ointment.)

▸ Sore throat lasts more than 5 days.

▸ Sinus congestion (fullness) lasts more than 14 days.

▸ Nasal discharge lasts more than 14 days.

▸ You have other questions or concerns.

Parent Care at Home If

▸ Mild cold with no complications.

Care Advice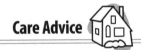

❶ What You Should Know About Colds

▪ It's normal for healthy children to get at least 6 colds a year. This is because so many viruses cause colds. With each new cold, your child's body builds up immunity to that virus.

▪ Most parents know when their child has a cold. Sometimes, they have it too or other children in school have it. Most often, you don't need to call or see your child's doctor. You do need to call your child's doctor if your child develops a complication. Examples are an earache or if the symptoms last too long.

▪ The normal cold lasts about 2 weeks. No medications make it go away sooner.

▪ There are good ways to help reduce many of the symptoms. With most colds, the starting symptom is a runny nose. This is followed in 3 or 4 days by a stuffy nose. Treatment for each symptom is different.

▪ Here is some care advice that should help.

❷ For a Runny Nose With Lots of Discharge: Blow or Suction the Nose

▪ Nasal mucus and discharge are washing germs out the nose and sinuses.

▪ Blowing the nose is all that's needed. Teach your child how to blow their nose at age 2 or 3 years.

- For younger children, gently suction the nose with a suction bulb.
- Put petroleum jelly on the skin under the nose. Wash the skin first with warm water. This will help protect the nostrils from any redness.

❸ Nasal Saline Rinse to Open a Blocked Nose

- Use saline (salt water) nose spray to loosen up dried mucus. If you don't have saline, you can use a few drops of water. Use distilled water, bottled water, or boiled tap water.
  - **Step 1.** Put 3 drops in each nostril. Age: If younger than 1 year, use 1 drop at a time.
  - **Step 2.** Blow (or suction) each nostril out while closing off the other nostril. Then, do the other side.
  - **Step 3.** Repeat nose drops and blowing (or suctioning) until the discharge is clear.
- **How often:** Do nasal saline rinses when your child can't breathe through the nose.
- **Age:** If younger than 1 year, no more than 4 times per day. Before breast or bottle-feedings is a good time.
- Saline nose drops or spray can be bought in any drugstore. No prescription is needed.
- **Reason for nose drops:** Suction or blowing alone can't remove dried or sticky mucus. Also, babies can't nurse or drink from a bottle unless the nose is open.
- **Other option:** Use a warm shower to loosen mucus. Breathe in the moist air and then blow each nostril.
- For young children, can also use a wet cotton swab to remove sticky mucus.

❹ Fluids: Offer More

- Try to get your child to drink lots of fluids.
- **Goal:** Keep your child well hydrated.
- It will also thin out mucus discharge from the nose.
- It also loosens up any phlegm in the lungs. Then it's easier to cough up.

❺ Humidifier

- If the air in your home is dry, use a humidifier.

- **Reason:** Dry air makes nasal mucus thicker.

❻ Medicines for Colds

- **Cold medicines.** Don't give any drugstore cold or cough medicines to young children. They are not approved by the US Food and Drug Administration for children younger than 6 years. (**Reason:** Not safe and can cause serious side effects.) Also, they are not helpful. (**Reason:** They can't remove dried mucus from the nose.) Nasal saline rinse works best.

- **Allergy medicines.** They are not helpful unless your child also has nasal allergies. They can also help an allergic cough.

- **No antibiotics.** Antibiotics are not helpful for colds. Antibiotics may be used if your child gets an ear or sinus infection.

❼ Other Symptoms of Colds: Treatment

- **Pain or fever.** Use acetaminophen (such as Tylenol) to treat muscle aches, sore throat, or headaches. Another choice is an ibuprofen product (such as Advil). You can also use these medicines for fever above 102°F (39°C).

- **Sore throat.** If older than 6 years, your child can also suck on hard candy. For children older than 1 year, sip warm chicken broth. Some children prefer cold foods such as Popsicles or ice cream.

- **Cough.** For children older than 1 year, give honey, ½ to 1 teaspoon (2.5–5 mL). (**Caution:** Do not use honey until 1 year of age.) If your child is older than 6 years, you can also use cough drops. Avoid cough drops before 6 years. (**Reason:** Risk of choking.)

- **Red eyes.** Rinse eyelids often with wet cotton balls.

❽ Return to School

- Your child can go back to school after the fever is gone. Your child should also feel well enough to join in normal activities. For practical purposes, the spread of colds can't be prevented.

❾ What to Expect

- Fever can last 2 to 3 days.

- Nasal drainage can last 7 to 14 days.

- Cough can last 2 to 3 weeks.

⑩ Call Your Doctor If

- Trouble breathing occurs.

- Earache occurs.

- Fever lasts more than 3 days or goes above 104°F (40°C).

- Any fever if younger than 12 weeks.

- Nasal discharge lasts more than 14 days.

- Cough lasts more than 3 weeks.

- You think your child needs to be seen.

- Your child becomes worse.

⑪ Extra Advice: Air Travel With Colds

- It's safe to fly when your child has a cold.

- She could get some mild ear congestion or even a brief earache while flying. Most often, that can be prevented. (See next advice [number 12].)

- Flying will not cause an ear infection.

⑫ Extra Advice: Prevent Ear Congestion During Air Travel

- Most symptoms happen when the airplane is coming down in altitude. This is the descent of the plane during the 15 minutes before landing.

- Keep your child awake during takeoff and descent.

- Have her swallow during descent using fluids or a pacifier.

- Children older than 4 years can chew gum during descent.

- Yawning during descent can also open the middle ear.

- Drink lots of fluids throughout the flight. This will prevent nasal secretions from drying out.

Remember!
Contact your doctor if your child develops any of the **Call Your Doctor** symptoms.

CHAPTER 16

Sinus Pain or Congestion

Definition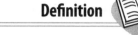

- Fullness, pressure, or pain on the face over a sinus.

- Sinus pain occurs above the eyebrow, behind the eye, and under the cheekbone.

- Other common symptoms include a blocked nose, nasal discharge, or postnasal drip.

See Other Chapter If

- **Age:** Younger than 5 years; does not sound like sinus congestion or pain. See Chapter 15, Colds.

- Nasal allergies cause the congestion. See Chapter 17, Nose Allergy (Hay Fever).

Symptoms

- Most often, the pain or pressure is on just one side of the face.

- Swelling around just one eye.

- Other common symptoms are a stuffy or blocked nose or nasal discharge. Your child may also have a nasal drip down the back of the throat. This is called a *postnasal drip.*

- Less common symptoms are bad breath or mouth breathing. Also, may have a sore throat and throat clearing from *postnasal drip.*

- Sinus pain is not a common symptom before 5 years of age.

Causes of Sinus Congestion

- **Viral sinus infection.** Part of the common cold. A cold infects lining of the nose. It also involves lining of all the sinuses.

- **Bacterial sinus infection.** A problem when the sinus becomes infected with bacteria. (Occurs in 5% of colds.) It starts as a viral sinus infection. Main symptoms are increased sinus pain and return of fever. Skin around the eyelids or cheeks may become red or swollen. Thick nasal secretions that last more than 14 days may point to a sinus infection. This can occur in younger children.

► **Allergic sinus reaction.** Sinus congestion often occurs with nasal allergies (such as from pollen). Sneezing, itchy nose, and clear nasal discharge point to this cause.

Treatment of Sinus Congestion

► **Viral sinus infection.** Nasal washes with saline. Antibiotics are not helpful.

► **Bacterial sinus infection.** Antibiotics by mouth.

► **Allergic sinus reaction.** Treatment of nasal allergy with allergy medicines often helps the sinus symptoms.

► **All thick nasal drainage.** Nasal secretions need treatment with nasal saline when they block the nose. Also, treat if they make breathing through the nose hard. If breathing is noisy, it may mean dried mucus is farther back. Nasal saline rinses can remove it.

Color of Nasal Discharge With Colds

► Nasal discharge changes color during different stages of a cold. This is normal.

► It starts as a clear discharge and later becomes cloudy.

► Sometimes it becomes yellow or green colored for a few days. This is still normal.

► Colored discharge is common after sleep, with allergy medicines, or with low humidity. (**Reason:** All of these events decrease the amount of normal nasal secretions.)

Bacterial Sinus Infections: When to Suspect

► Yellow or green nasal discharge is seen with both viral and bacterial sinus infections. Suspect a bacterial infection if the discharge becomes thick (like pus). But, it also needs one or more of the following symptoms:

• Sinus pain, not just normal sinus congestion. Pain occurs mainly behind the cheekbone or eye.

• Swelling or redness of the skin over any sinus.

• Fever lasts more than 3 days.

• Fever returns after it's been gone for more than 24 hours.

• Nasal discharge and postnasal drip lasts more than 14 days without improvement.

When to Call Your Doctor

Call 911 Now (Your Child May Need an Ambulance) If

▶ Not moving or too weak to stand.

▶ Severe trouble breathing (struggling for each breath, can barely speak or cry).

▶ You think your child has a life-threatening emergency.

Go to ER Now If

▶ Acts or talks confused.

Call Your Doctor Now (Night or Day) If

▶ Trouble breathing, but not severe. (**Exception**: Gone after cleaning out the nose.)

▶ Redness or swelling on the cheek or forehead or around the eye.

▶ Severe headache and becomes worse.

▶ Severe pain and not better after using this chapter's Care Advice.

▶ Weak immune system (such as sickle cell disease, HIV, cancer, organ transplant, or taking oral steroids).

▶ Fever higher than 104°F (40°C).

▶ Your child looks or acts very sick.

▶ You think your child needs to be seen, and the problem is urgent.

Call Your Doctor Within 24 Hours If

▶ Headache lasts more than 48 hours.

▶ Fever lasts more than 3 days.

▶ Fever returns after being gone for more than 24 hours.

▶ Earache occurs.

▶ Sinus pain with fever.

▶ You think your child needs to be seen, but the problem is not urgent.

Call Your Doctor During Weekday Office Hours If

▶ Sinus pain still there after using nasal washes and pain medicine for 24 hours.

▶ Thick yellow or green pus draining from nose and not improved by nasal washes. (**Exception:** Yellow or green tinged secretions are normal.)

▶ Sinus congestion and fullness lasts more than 2 weeks.

▸ Nasal discharge lasts more than 2 weeks.

▸ You have other questions or concerns.

Parent Care at Home If

▸ Normal sinus congestion as part of a cold.

Care Advice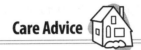

❶ What You Should Know About Sinus Congestion

■ Sinus congestion is a normal part of a cold.

■ Nasal discharge normally changes color during different stages of a cold. It starts as clear, turns cloudy, then turns yellow or green tinged, and then dries up.

■ Yellow- or green-tinged discharge. This is more common with sleep, antihistamines, or low humidity. (**Reason:** Decreases the amount of normal nasal secretions.)

■ Usually, nasal washes can prevent a bacterial sinus infection.

■ Antibiotics are not helpful for sinus congestion that occurs with colds.

■ Here is some care advice that should help.

❷ Nasal Saline Rinse to Open a Blocked Nose

■ Use saline (salt water) nose spray (such as store brand) to loosen up dried mucus. If you don't have saline, you can use a few drops of water. Use bottled water, distilled water, or boiled tap water. Teens can just splash a little water in the nose and then blow.

  – **Step 1.** Put 3 drops in each nostril.

  – **Step 2.** Blow each nostril out while closing off the other nostril. Then, do the other side.

  – **Step 3.** Repeat nose drops and blowing until the discharge is clear.

■ **How often:** Do saline rinses when your child can't breathe through the nose.

■ Saline nose drops or spray can be bought in any drugstore. No prescription is needed.

- **Reason for nose drops:** Suction or blowing alone can't remove dried or sticky mucus.

- **Other option:** Use a warm shower to loosen mucus. Breathe in the moist air and then blow each nostril.

❸ Fluids: Offer More

- Try to get your child to drink lots of fluids.

- **Goal:** Keep your child well hydrated.

- It will also thin out mucus discharge from the nose.

- It also loosens up any phlegm in the lungs. Then it's easier to cough up.

❹ Humidifier

- If the air in your home is dry, use a humidifier. (**Reason:** Dry air makes nasal mucus thicker.)

❺ Decongestant Nose Spray (Age: 12 Years or Older)

- Use this only if the sinus still seems blocked after nasal washes. Use the long-acting type (such as Afrin).

- **Dose:** 1 spray on each side. Do this 2 times per day.

- Always clean out the nose before using.

- Use for 1 day. After that, use only for symptoms.

- Don't use for more than 3 days. (**Reason:** Can cause rebound congestion.)

- Decongestants given by mouth (such as Sudafed) are another choice. They can also open a stuffy nose and ears. Side effects: They may make a person feel nervous or dizzy. Follow the package directions.

❻ Pain Medicine

- To help with pain, give an acetaminophen product (such as Tylenol).

- Another choice is an ibuprofen product (such as Advil).

- Use as needed.

❼ Cold Pack for Pain

- For pain or swelling, use a cold pack. You can also use ice wrapped in a wet cloth.

- Put it over the sinus for 20 minutes.

- **Caution:** Avoid frostbite.

❽ Allergy Medicine

- If your child also has nasal allergies, give an allergy medicine. Long-acting allergy medicines (such as Zyrtec) are best. (**Reason:** These medicines do not cause your child to act sleepy. Age limit: 2 years and older.)

- A single dose of Benadryl can be given for any breakthrough symptoms. Age limit: 1 year and older.

- No prescription is needed.

❾ What to Expect

- With this advice, viral sinus blockage goes away in 7 to 14 days.

- The main problem is a sinus infection from bacteria. This can occur if bacteria multiply within the blocked sinus. This leads to a fever and increased pain. It needs antibiotics. Once treated, symptoms will improve in a few days.

❿ Return to School

- Sinus infections cannot be spread to others.

- Your child can return to school after the fever is gone. Your child should feel well enough to join in normal activities.

⓫ Call Your Doctor If

- Sinus pain lasts more than 24 hours after starting treatment.

- Sinus congestion lasts more than 2 weeks.

- Fever lasts more than 3 days.

- You think your child needs to be seen.

- Your child becomes worse.

Remember!
Contact your doctor if your child develops any of the **Call Your Doctor** symptoms.

CHAPTER 17

Nose Allergy (Hay Fever)

Definition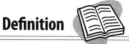

▶ An allergic reaction of the nose, usually due to pollen.

▶ An itchy nose, clear discharge, and sneezing.

See Other Chapter If

▶ Does not look like hay fever. See Chapter 15, Colds.

Triggers of Nasal Allergies

▶ **Cause.** An allergic reaction of the nose and sinuses to an inhaled substance. The medical name for this is *allergic rhinitis*. The allergic substance is called an *allergen*. Most allergens float in the air. That's how they get in the nose. Here are the common ones.

• **Pollens.** Trees, grass, weeds, and molds are the most common pollens. Tree pollens arrive in the spring. Grass pollens appear in the summer. Weed pollens come in the fall. Pollens cause seasonal allergies. You can't avoid pollens because they are in the air. Most nasal allergies continue through pollen season. They can last 4 to 8 weeks. Pollens cause seasonal allergic rhinitis. This is also called *hay fever.*

• **Pets.** Allergens can also be from cats, dogs, horses, rabbits, and other animals. Most people don't keep a pet that they are allergic to. They will only have sporadic allergy symptoms when they are exposed to that specific animal. These symptoms will usually last a few hours. If someone with a cat visits, they will bring cat dander with them. This will cause brief symptoms. If you own the pet, though, your child will have symptoms all the time.

• **House dust.** House dust contains many allergens. It always contains dust mites. If your humidity is high, it will contain mold. House dust causes year-round, daily symptoms. The medical name for this is *perennial allergic rhinitis.*

Symptoms of Nasal Allergies

- Clear nasal discharge with sneezing, sniffing, and itching of nose (in 100% of children).

- Eye allergies (itchy, red, watery, and puffy) can also occur (70%).

- Ear and sinus congestion or fullness can occur.

- Throat can also feel scratchy or have a tickly feeling at times.

- Itchy ear canals, itchy skin, or hoarse voice sometimes also occur.

How to Tell Seasonal Nasal Allergies From the Common Cold

- Symptoms happen during pollen season.

- Had the same symptoms during the same month last year.

- Hay fever symptoms last 6 to 8 weeks for each pollen. (Colds last 1–3 weeks.)

- Allergies: Itchy eyes and nose. Not seen with colds.

- Colds: Fever and/or sore throat. Not seen with allergies.

- Both: Runny nose and watery eyes. Can also have a cough with both, but less common with allergies.

Nose and Eye Allergies: Age of Onset

- Seasonal pollen allergies usually begin at age 2 to 5 years.

- Symptoms peak in school-aged children, teens, and young adults.

- Pollen symptoms are rare in children younger than 2 years. They require at least 2 seasons of exposure to the pollen.

- Children younger than 2 who have chronic nasal symptoms have other causes. Examples are recurrent colds, large adenoids, or cow's milk allergy.

- Food allergies can start during the first year of life, but not pollen allergies.

When to Call Your Doctor

Call Your Doctor Within 24 Hours If

- You think your child needs to be seen.

- Lots of coughing.

- Sinus pain (not just congestion) does not go away with allergy medicines. (**Note:** Sinus pain is around the cheekbone or eyes.)

Call Your Doctor During Weekday Office Hours If

▶ Hay fever symptoms make it hard to go to school or do normal activities. (**Note:** Taking allergy medicine for 2 days has not helped.)

▶ Diagnosis of hay fever has never been made by a doctor.

▶ Year-round symptoms of nasal allergies.

▶ Snoring is a frequent problem.

▶ You have other questions or concerns.

Parent Care at Home If

▶ Nasal allergy symptoms or hay fever.

Care Advice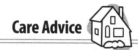

❶ What You Should Know About Nose Allergies or Hay Fever

▪ Hay fever is very common. It happens in about 15% of children.

▪ Nose and eye symptoms can be controlled by giving allergy medicines.

▪ Pollens are in the air every day during pollen season, so allergy medicines must be given daily. They need to be used for 2 months or longer during pollen season.

▪ Here is some care advice that should help.

❷ Allergy Medicines

▪ Allergy medicines are called *antihistamines*. They are the drug of choice for nasal allergies.

▪ They will help control the symptoms. These include a runny nose, nasal itching, and sneezing.

▪ The key to control is to give allergy medicine every day during pollen season.

❸ Long-Acting Allergy Medicines

▪ Long-acting allergy medicine (such as Zyrtec) is best for nasal allergies. No prescription is needed. Age limit: 2 years or older.

▪ **Advantage:** Causes less sedation than older allergy medicine such as Benadryl. It is long acting and lasts up to 24 hours.

- **Dose:** Follow the package directions.

  - **Downside:** Sometimes will have breakthrough symptoms before 24 hours. If that happens, you can give a single dose of Benadryl. Age limit: 1 year and older.

  - **Cost:** Ask the pharmacist for a store brand. (**Reason:** Costs less than the brand-name products.)

➍ Nasal Saline Rinse to Wash Out Pollen

- Use saline (salt water) nose drops or spray (such as store brand). This helps wash out pollen or loosen up dried mucus. If you don't have saline, you can use a few drops of water. Use bottled water, distilled water, or boiled tap water. Teens can just splash a little water in the nose and then blow.

  - **Step 1.** Put 3 drops in each nostril.

  - **Step 2.** Blow each nostril out while closing off the other nostril. Then, do the other side.

  - **Step 3.** Repeat nose drops and blowing until the discharge is clear.

- **How often:** Do nasal saline rinses when your child can't breathe through the nose. Also, do them if the nose is very itchy.

- Saline nose drops or spray can be bought in any drugstore. No prescription is needed.

- Saline nose drops can also be made at home. Use ½ teaspoon (2.5 mL) of table salt. Stir the salt into 1 cup (8 ounces or 240 mL) of warm water. Use bottled or boiled water to make saline nose drops.

- **Other option:** Use a warm shower to loosen mucus. Breathe in the moist air and then blow each nostril.

➎ Eye Allergy Treatment

- For eye symptoms, wash off the face and eyelids. This will remove pollen or any other allergic substances.

- Then put a cold, wet washcloth on the eyes.

- Most often, an allergy medicine given by mouth will help eye symptoms. Sometimes, eyedrops are also needed. (See next advice [numbers 6 and 7].)

❻ Antihistamine Eyedrops (Ketotifen) for Eye Allergy Symptoms: First Choice

- Ketotifen eyedrops (such as Zaditor) are a safe and effective product. No prescription is needed.
- **Dose:** 1 drop every 12 hours.
- For severe allergies, use ketotifen eyedrops every day during pollen season. This will give the best control.

❼ Antihistamine/Vasoconstrictive Eyedrops for Eye Allergy Symptoms: Second Choice

- Ask your pharmacist to suggest a brand (such as Visine-A). The *A* stands for antihistamine. No prescription is needed.
- **Dose:** 1 drop every 8 hours.
- Do not use for more than 5 days. (**Reason:** Will cause red eyes from rebound effect.)
- **Downside:** Doesn't work as well as Ketotifen eyedrops.

❽ Wash Pollen Off Body

- Remove pollen from the hair and skin with shampoo and a shower. This is especially important before bedtime.

❾ What to Expect

- Since pollen allergies recur each year, learn to control the symptoms.

❿ Pollen: How to Reduce the Pollen Your Child Breathes

- Pollen is carried in the air.
- Keep windows closed in the home, at least in your child's bedroom.
- Keep windows closed in car. Turn the air conditioner on recirculate.
- Avoid window or attic fans. They pull in pollen.
- Try to stay indoors on windy days. (**Reason:** The pollen count is much higher when it's dry and windy.)
- Avoid playing with outdoor pets. (**Reason:** Pollen collects in the fur.)
- **Pollen count:** You can get your daily pollen count from **www.pollen.com**. Just type in your zip code.

⓫ Call Your Doctor If

- Symptoms are not better in 2 days after starting allergy medicine.
- You think your child needs to be seen.
- Your child becomes worse.

Remember!
Contact your doctor if your child develops any of the **Call Your Doctor** symptoms.

CHAPTER 18

Nosebleed

Definition

► Bleeding from 1 or both nostrils.

► Nosebleeds not caused by an injury.

Causes of Nosebleeds

► Nosebleeds are common because of the rich blood supply of the nose. Common causes include

- **Spontaneous nosebleed.** Most nosebleeds start without a known cause.

- **Rubbing.** Rubbing or picking the nose is the most common known cause. It's hard to not touch or rub the nose.

- **Blowing.** Blowing the nose too hard can cause a nose bleed.

- **Suctioning.** Suctioning the nose can sometimes cause bleeding. This can happen if the suction tip is put in too far.

- **Sinus infections.** The main symptoms are lots of dry nasal discharge and a blocked nose. This leads to extra nose blowing and picking. The sinus infection is more often viral than bacterial.

- **Nose allergies.** The main symptom is a very itchy nose. This leads to extra rubbing and blowing, which could lead to bleeding.

- **Dry air.** Dryness of the nasal lining makes it more likely to bleed. In the winter, forced air heating can often dry out the nose.

- **Allergy medicines.** These help the nasal symptoms but also dry out the nose.

- **Ibuprofen and aspirin.** These medicines increase bleeding tendency. Aspirin is not used in children.

- **Bleeding disorder (serious).** This means the blood platelets or clotting factors are missing or not working right. A bleeding disorder should be suspected if the nosebleed can't be stopped. Excessive bleeding from the gums or with minor cuts is also a clue. Bleeding disorders are a rare cause of frequent nosebleeds.

When to Call Your Doctor

Call 911 Now (Your Child May Need an Ambulance) If

- ▶ Passed out (fainted) or too weak to stand.
- ▶ You think your child has a life-threatening emergency.

Go to ER Now If

- ▶ Bleeding a lot after 20 minutes of squeezing the nose correctly.

Call Your Doctor Now (Night or Day) If

- ▶ Nosebleed that won't stop after 10 minutes of squeezing the nose correctly.
- ▶ Large amount of blood has been lost.
- ▶ New skin bruises or bleeding gums not caused by an injury also present.
- ▶ High-risk child (such as with low platelets or other bleeding disorder).
- ▶ You think your child needs to be seen, and the problem is urgent.

Call Your Doctor Within 24 Hours If

- ▶ You think your child needs to be seen, but the problem is not urgent.

Call Your Doctor During Weekday Office Hours If

- ▶ **Age:** Younger than 1 year.
- ▶ New-onset nosebleeds happen 3 or more times in a week.
- ▶ Hard-to-stop nosebleeds are a frequent problem.
- ▶ Easy bleeding is present in other family members.
- ▶ You have other questions or concerns.

Parent Care at Home If

- ▶ Mild nosebleed.

Care Advice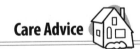

❶ What You Should Know About Nosebleeds

- ■ Nosebleeds are common.
- ■ You should be able to stop the bleeding if you use the correct technique.
- ■ Here is some care advice that should help.

❷ Squeeze the Lower Nose

- Use the thumb and index finger in a pinching manner.

- Gently squeeze soft parts of the lower nose together and lean head forward. Press them against the center wall of the nose for 10 minutes. This puts constant pressure on the bleeding point.

- If bleeding continues, move your point of pressure.

- Have your child sit up and breathe through the mouth during this procedure.

- If the nose rebleeds, use the same technique again.

❸ Put Gauze Into the Nose

- If pressure alone fails, use a piece of gauze. Wet it with a few drops of water. Another option is to put a little petroleum jelly (such as Vaseline) on it. Insert the wet gauze into the side that is bleeding. Press again for 10 minutes. (**Reason:** This works because gauze puts more pressure on the bleeding spot.)

- Special nose drops: If your child has lots of nosebleeds, buy some decongestant nose drops. An example is Afrin. No prescription is needed. Place 3 drops on the gauze and press as above. These nose drops shrink the blood vessels in the nose. (**Caution:** Don't use decongestant nose drops if your child is younger than 1 year.)

- If you don't have gauze, use a piece of paper towel.

- Repeat the process of gently squeezing the lower soft parts of the nose. Do this for 10 minutes.

❹ Prevent Recurrent Nosebleeds

- If the air in your home is dry, use a humidifier to keep the nose from drying out.

- For nose blowing, blow gently.

- For nose suctioning, don't put the suction tip very far inside. Also, move it gently.

- Do not use aspirin and ibuprofen. (**Reason:** Increases bleeding tendency.)

- Bleeding areas in the front of the nose sometimes develop a scab. It may heal slowly and rebleed. If that happens to your child, try this tip: Apply a small amount of petroleum jelly (such as Vaseline) to the spot. Repeat twice a day. Do not use for more than 1 week.

❺ What to Expect

- More than 99% of nosebleeds will stop if you press on the right spot.

- It may take 10 minutes of direct pressure.

- After swallowing blood from a nosebleed, your child may vomit or cough up a little blood.

- Your child may also pass a dark stool tomorrow because of swallowed blood.

❻ Call Your Doctor If

- Can't stop bleeding with 10 minutes of direct pressure done correctly.

- You think your child needs to be seen.

- Your child becomes worse.

Remember!
Contact your doctor if your child develops any of the **Call Your Doctor** symptoms.

PART 6

Mouth or Throat Symptoms

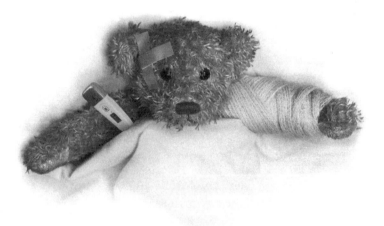

CHAPTER 19

Sore Throat

Definition

► Pain or discomfort of the throat.

► Made worse with swallowing.

► Not caused by an injury to the throat.

See Other Chapter If

► Main symptom is croup. See Chapter 27, Croup.

► Main symptom is cough. See Chapter 26, Cough.

► After an injury to the throat. See Chapter 23, Mouth Injury.

Causes of Sore Throat

► **Colds.** Most sore throats are part of a cold. In fact, a sore throat may be the only symptom for the first 24 hours. Then a cough and runny nose occur.

► **Viral pharyngitis.** Some viruses cause a sore throat without other symptoms. A cough and runny nose don't become part of the illness. An antibiotic won't help.

► **Strep pharyngitis (strep throat).** Group A strep infection is the most common bacterial cause. It accounts for 20% of sore throats without any cold symptoms. Pus is seen on the tonsils. Peak age is 5 to 15 years. An antibiotic is helpful.

► **Infectious mononucleosis ("mono").** Mainly occurs in teens and young adults. Main symptoms are sore throat, fever, and widespread swollen lymph nodes. Like strep throat, mono also has pus on the tonsils. Patients with mono may also have a large spleen. It's located in the upper left side of the stomach. Mono is diagnosed with special blood tests.

► **Postnasal drip.** Drainage from a sinus infection can cause a sore throat. Throat clearing that goes with the drainage may cause most of the irritation. Sinus infection is more likely to be viral than bacterial.

► **Mouth breathing.** Breathing with the mouth open during sleep can cause a sore throat. After eating breakfast, it often goes away.

▸ **Abscess of tonsil (serious).** A bacterial infection of the tonsil can spread to surrounding tissues. Main symptoms are severe trouble swallowing, fever, and one-sided throat pain. It's also hard to fully open the mouth. The peak age is the teen years.

▸ **Epiglottitis (very serious).** A bacterial infection of the flap of tissue above the vocal cords. It normally covers the windpipe during swallowing. Main symptoms are severe sore throat, drooling, spitting, and fever. It can shut off the airway. Needs a 911 response. Fortunately, epiglottitis is nearly unheard of in fully vaccinated children.

Strep Throat: When to Suspect It

▸ Symptoms include sore throat, fever, headache, stomach pain, nausea, and vomiting.

▸ Cough, hoarseness, red eyes, and runny nose are usually not seen with strep throat. These symptoms point more to a viral cause.

▸ Scarlet fever rash (fine, red or pink, sandpaper-like rash) is highly suggestive of strep throat.

▸ Peak age: 5 to 15 years. Not common in babies and children younger than 2 years unless a sibling has strep throat.

▸ If you think your child has strep throat, call your doctor.

▸ Your doctor will do a strep test. If the test is positive for *Strep*, your doctor will start treatment. There is no risk from waiting until a strep test can be done.

▸ Standard treatment is with antibiotics by mouth.

Symptoms in Babies and Toddlers

▸ Babies and children younger than 2 years usually don't report a sore throat. A young child who does not want favorite foods may have a sore throat. He may also start to cry during feedings.

When to Call Your Doctor

Call 911 Now (Your Child May Need an Ambulance) If

▸ Severe trouble breathing (struggling for each breath, can barely speak or cry).

▸ Purple or blood-colored spots or dots on skin with fever.

▸ You think your child has a life-threatening emergency.

Go to ER Now If

▶ Can't swallow any fluids and new-onset drooling.

▶ Purple or blood-colored spots or dots on skin without fever.

Call Your Doctor Now (Night or Day) If

▶ Trouble breathing, but not severe.

▶ Great trouble swallowing fluids or spit.

▶ Can't open mouth all the way.

▶ Stiff neck or can't move neck normally.

▶ Dehydration suspected (no urine in more than 8 hours, dark urine, very dry mouth, and no tears).

▶ Weak immune system (such as sickle cell disease, HIV, cancer, organ transplant, or taking oral steroids).

▶ Fever above 104°F (40°C).

▶ Your child looks or acts very sick.

▶ You think your child needs to be seen, and the problem is urgent. (**Note:** A strep test is not urgent.)

Call Your Doctor Within 24 Hours If

▶ Sore throat pain is severe and doesn't improve 2 hours after taking ibuprofen.

▶ Large lymph nodes in the neck.

▶ Pink rash that's widespread.

▶ Earache or ear discharge.

▶ Sinus pain (not just congestion) around cheekbone or eyes.

▶ Fever lasts more than 3 days.

▶ Fever returns after being gone for more than 24 hours.

▶ **Age:** Younger than 2 years.

▶ Close contact to a person with strep throat within the last 7 days.

▶ Sores on the skin.

▶ You think your child needs to be seen, but the problem is not urgent. (Or needs a strep test.)

Call Your Doctor During Weekday Office Hours If

▸ Sore throat is the main symptom and lasts more than 48 hours.

▸ Sore throat with cold/cough symptoms lasts more than 5 days.

▸ You have other questions or concerns.

Parent Care at Home If

▸ Viral throat infection suspected.

Care Advice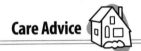

❶ What You Should Know About Sore Throats

■ Most sore throats are just part of a cold and caused by a virus.

■ A cough, hoarse voice, or nasal discharge points to a cold as the cause.

■ Most children with a sore throat don't need to see their doctor.

■ Here is some care advice that should help.

❷ Sore Throat Pain Relief

■ **Age:** Older than 1 year. Can sip warm fluids, such as chicken broth or apple juice. Some children prefer cold foods such as Popsicles or ice cream.

■ **Age:** Older than 6 years. Can also suck on hard candy or lollipops. Butterscotch seems to help.

■ **Age:** Older than 8 years. Can also gargle. Use warm water with a little table salt added. A liquid antacid can be added instead of salt. Use Mylanta or the store brand. No prescription is needed.

■ Medicated throat sprays or lozenges are generally not helpful.

❸ Pain Medicine

■ To help with pain, give an acetaminophen product (such as Tylenol).

■ Another choice is an ibuprofen product (such as Advil).

■ Use as needed.

❹ Fever Medicine

■ For fevers above 102°F (39°C), give an acetaminophen product (such as Tylenol).

■ Another choice is an ibuprofen product (such as Advil).

- **Note:** Fevers under 102°F (39°C) are important for fighting infections.
- **For all fevers:** Keep your child well hydrated. Give lots of cold fluids.

❺ Fluids and Soft Diet

- Try to get your child to drink adequate fluids.
- **Goal:** Keep your child well hydrated. Cold drinks, milk shakes, Popsicles, slushes, and sherbet are good choices.
- **Solid foods:** Offer a soft diet. Also, avoid foods that need a lot of chewing. Avoid citrus, salty, or spicy foods. (**Note:** Fluid intake is much more important than eating any solid foods.)
- Swollen tonsils can make some solid foods hard to swallow. Cut food into smaller pieces.

❻ Return to School

- Your child can return to school after the fever is gone. Your child should feel well enough to join in normal activities.
- Most often, having just a sore throat is not a reason to miss school.
- Children with strep throat need to be taking an antibiotic for 12 hours.

❼ What to Expect

- Most often, sore throats with a viral illness last 4 or 5 days.

❽ Call Your Doctor If

- Sore throat is the main symptom and lasts more than 48 hours.
- Sore throat with a cold lasts more than 5 days.
- Fever lasts more than 3 days or goes above 104°F (40°C).
- You think your child needs to be seen.
- Your child becomes worse.

Remember!
Contact your doctor if your child develops any of the **Call Your Doctor** symptoms.

CHAPTER 20

Strep Throat Infection

Definition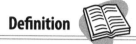

▸ Your child was diagnosed with a strep throat infection.

▸ A doctor has told you your child probably has strep throat OR

▸ Your child has a positive strep test.

▸ Your child is taking an antibiotic for strep throat and you have questions.

▸ You are worried that the fever or sore throat is not getting better fast enough.

See Other Chapter If

▸ Sore throat is present, but you have not been told your child has strep throat. See Chapter 19, Sore Throat.

Symptoms of Strep Throat Infection

▸ Pain or discomfort of the throat.

▸ Pain is made worse with swallowing.

▸ Babies and children younger than 2 years usually can't report a sore throat. A young child who does not want favorite foods may have a sore throat. She may also start to cry during feedings.

▸ Other symptoms include sore throat, fever, headache, stomach pain, nausea, and vomiting.

▸ Cough, hoarseness, red eyes, and runny nose are not seen with strep throat. These symptoms point more to a viral cause.

▸ Scarlet fever rash (fine, red or pink, sandpaper-like rash) is highly suggestive of strep throat.

▸ If you look at the throat with a light, it will be bright red. The tonsils will be red and swollen, often covered with pus.

▸ Peak age: 5 to 15 years. Not common in babies and children younger than 2 years unless a sibling has strep throat.

Cause of Strep Throat

▸ Group A *Strep* is the only common bacterial cause of a throat infection. The medical name for strep throat is *strep pharyngitis.*

▸ It accounts for 20% of sore throats with fever.

▸ Any infection of the throat usually also involves the tonsils. The medical name is *strep tonsillitis.*

Diagnosis of Strep Throat

▸ Diagnosis can be confirmed by a strep test on a sample of throat secretions.

▸ There is no risk in waiting until a strep test can be done.

▸ If your child has cold symptoms too, a strep test is usually not needed.

Prevention of Spread to Others

▸ Good hand washing can prevent spread of infection.

When to Call Your Doctor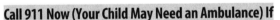

Call 911 Now (Your Child May Need an Ambulance) If

▸ Severe trouble breathing (struggling for each breath, can barely speak or cry).

▸ Fainted or too weak to stand.

▸ Purple or blood-colored spots or dots on skin with fever.

▸ You think your child has a life-threatening emergency.

Go to ER Now If

▸ Can't swallow any fluids and new-onset drooling.

▸ Purple or blood-colored spots or dots on skin without fever.

Call Your Doctor Now (Night or Day) If

▸ Trouble breathing, but not severe.

▸ Great trouble swallowing fluids or saliva.

▸ Stiff neck or can't move neck like normal.

▸ Dehydration suspected (no urine in over 8 hours, dark urine, very dry mouth, and no tears).

▸ Fever above 104°F (40°C).

- Will not drink or drinks very little for more than 8 hours.

- Can't open mouth all the way.

- Your child looks or acts very sick.

- You think your child needs to be seen, and the problem is urgent.

Call Your Doctor Within 24 Hours If

- Urine is pink or tea (brown) colored.

- Taking antibiotic more than 24 hours, and sore throat pain is severe. (The pain is not better 2 hours after taking pain medicines.)

- Taking antibiotic more than 48 hours and fever still present or comes back.

- Taking antibiotic more than 3 days and other strep throat symptoms not better.

- You think your child needs to be seen, but the problem is not urgent.

Call Your Doctor During Weekday Office Hours If

- You have other questions or concerns.

Parent Care at Home If

- Strep throat infection on antibiotic with no complications.

Care Advice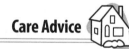

❶ What You Should Know About Strep Throat

- *Strep* causes 20% of throat and tonsil infections in school-aged children.

- Viral infections cause the rest.

- Strep throat is easy to treat with an antibiotic.

- Complications are rare.

- Here is some care advice that should help.

❷ Antibiotic by Mouth

- Strep throat infections need a prescription for an antibiotic.

- The antibiotic will kill bacteria that are causing the strep throat infection.

- Give the antibiotic as directed.

- Try not to forget any doses.

- Give the antibiotic until it is gone. (**Reason:** To stop strep throat infection from flaring up again.)

❸ Sore Throat Pain Relief

- **Age:** Older than 1 year. Can sip warm fluids, such as chicken broth or apple juice. Some children prefer cold foods such as Popsicles or ice cream.
- **Age:** Older than 6 years. Can also suck on hard candy or lollipops. Butterscotch seems to help.
- **Age:** Older than 8 years. Can also gargle. Use warm water with a little table salt added. A liquid antacid can be added instead of salt. Use Mylanta or the store brand. No prescription is needed.
- Medicated throat sprays or lozenges are generally not helpful.

❹ Pain Medicine

- To help with pain, give an acetaminophen product (such as Tylenol).
- Another choice is an ibuprofen product (such as Advil).
- Use as needed.

❺ Fever Medicine

- For fevers above 102°F (39°C), give an acetaminophen product (such as Tylenol).
- Another choice is an ibuprofen product (such as Advil).
- **Note:** Fevers under 102°F (39°C) are important for fighting infections.
- **For all fevers:** Keep your child well hydrated. Give lots of cold fluids.

❻ Fluids and Soft Diet

- Try to get your child to drink adequate fluids.
- **Goal:** Keep your child well hydrated.
- Cold drinks, milk shakes, Popsicles, slushes, and sherbet are good choices.
- **Solids:** Offer a soft diet. Also, avoid foods that need a lot of chewing. Avoid citrus, salty, or spicy foods. (**Note:** Fluid intake is much more important than eating any solids.)
- Swollen tonsils can make some solid foods hard to swallow. Cut food into smaller pieces.

❼ What to Expect

- Strep throat responds quickly to antibiotics.
- The fever is usually gone within 24 hours.
- The sore throat starts to feel better within 48 hours.

❽ Return to School

- Your child can return to school after the fever is gone.
- Your child should feel well enough to join in normal activities.
- Children with strep throat need to be taking an antibiotic for at least 12 hours.

❾ Call Your Doctor If

- Trouble breathing or drooling occurs.
- Dehydration suspected.
- Fever lasts more than 2 days after starting antibiotics.
- Sore throat lasts more than 3 days after starting antibiotics.
- You think your child needs to be seen.
- Your child becomes worse.

Remember!
Contact your doctor if your child develops any of the **Call Your Doctor** symptoms.

CHAPTER 21

Lymph Nodes, Swollen

Definition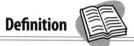

- ▸ Increased size of 1 or more lymph nodes.
- ▸ Most are in the neck.
- ▸ Also includes swollen lymph nodes in the armpit or groin.
- ▸ The lymph node is larger than the same node on the other side of the body.
- ▸ Normal nodes are usually less than ½ in (1.3 cm) across. This is the size of a pea or baked bean.

See Other Chapter If

- ▸ Swollen node is in the neck and your child has a sore throat. See Chapter 19, Sore Throat.

Causes of Swollen Lymph Nodes

- ▸ **Neck nodes.** Cervical (neck) nodes are most commonly involved. This is because many types of respiratory tract infections occur during childhood.

- ▸ **Viral throat infection.** This is the most common cause of swollen nodes in the neck. The swollen nodes are usually ½ to 1 in (1.3–2.5 cm) across. They are the same on each side.

- ▸ **Bacterial throat infection.** A swollen node with a bacterial throat infection is usually just on one side. It can be quite large—over 1 in or 2.5 cm across. This is about the size of a quarter. Most often, it's the node that drains the tonsil.

- ▸ **Tooth decay or abscess.** This causes a swollen, tender node under the jawbone. Only one node is involved. The lower face may also be swollen on that side.

- ▸ **Armpit swollen nodes.** Causes include skin infections (such as impetigo) and a rash (such as poison ivy).

- ▸ **Groin swollen nodes.** Causes include skin infections (such as athlete's foot) and a retained foreign object (such as a sliver).

- ▸ **Shaving.** Teen girls can cause low-grade infections when shaving the legs.

▸ **Widespread swollen nodes.** Swollen nodes everywhere suggest an infection spread in the blood. An example is infectious mononucleosis ("mono"). Widespread rashes such as eczema can also cause all nodes to enlarge.

▸ **Normal nodes.** Lymph nodes can always be felt in the neck and groin. They are about the size of a bean. They never go away.

Lymph Nodes: What They Drain

▸ Lymph nodes are filled with white blood cells. They filter the lymph fluid coming from certain parts of the body. They fight infections.

▸ **Neck nodes in front.** These drain the nose, throat, and lower face.

▸ **Neck nodes in back.** These drain the scalp.

▸ **Armpit nodes.** These drain the arms and upper chest wall.

▸ **Groin nodes.** These drain the legs and lower stomach wall.

Common Objects Used to Guess the Size

▸ **Pea or pencil eraser:** ¼ in or 6 mm.

▸ **Dime:** ¾ in or 1.9 cm.

▸ **Quarter:** 1 in or 2.5 cm.

▸ **Golf ball:** 1½ in or 3.8 cm.

▸ **Tennis ball:** 2½ in or 6.4 cm.

When to Call Your Doctor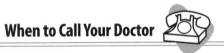

Call Your Doctor Now (Night or Day) If

▸ Node in the neck causes trouble with breathing, swallowing, or drinking.

▸ Fever above 104°F (40°C).

▸ Skin over the node is red.

▸ Node gets much bigger within 6 hours or less.

▸ Your child looks or acts very sick.

▸ You think your child needs to be seen, and the problem is urgent.

Call Your Doctor Within 24 Hours If

▸ Measures 1 in (2.5 cm) or more in size.

▸ Very tender to the touch.

- ▶ **Age:** Younger than 3 months.
- ▶ Node limits moving the neck, arm, or leg.
- ▶ Toothache with a swollen node under the jawbone.
- ▶ Fever lasts more than 3 days.
- ▶ You think your child needs to be seen, but the problem is not urgent.

Call Your Doctor During Weekday Office Hours If

- ▶ Node in the neck and also has a sore throat.
- ▶ Large nodes at 2 or more parts of the body.
- ▶ Cause of the swollen node is not clear.
- ▶ Large node lasts more than 1 month.
- ▶ You have other questions or concerns.

Parent Care at Home If

- ▶ Mildly swollen lymph node.

Care Advice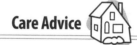

❶ What You Should Know About Normal Nodes

- ▪ If you have found a pea- or bean-sized node, this is normal. Normal lymph nodes are smaller than ½ in or 1.3 cm.
- ▪ Don't look for lymph nodes because you can almost always find some. They are easy to find in the neck and groin.

❷ What You Should Know About Swollen Nodes From a Viral Infection

- ▪ Viral throat infections and colds can cause lymph nodes in the neck to grow bigger. They may double in size. They may also become tender.
- ▪ This reaction is normal. It means the lymph node is fighting the infection and doing a good job.
- ▪ Here is some care advice that should help.

❸ Pain Medicine

- ▪ To help with pain, give an acetaminophen product (such as Tylenol).
- ▪ Another choice is an ibuprofen product (such as Advil).
- ▪ Use as needed.

❹ Fever Medicine

- For fevers above 102°F (39°C), give an acetaminophen product (such as Tylenol).
- Another choice is an ibuprofen product (such as Advil).
- **Note:** Fevers under 102°F (39°C) are important for fighting infections.
- **For all fevers:** Keep your child well hydrated. Give lots of cold fluids.

❺ Do Not Squeeze

- Don't squeeze lymph nodes.
- **Reason:** This may keep them from shrinking back to normal size.

❻ Return to School

- Swollen lymph nodes alone cannot be spread to others.
- If the swollen nodes are caused by a viral illness, your child can return to school. Wait until after the fever is gone. Your child should feel well enough to participate in normal activities.

❼ What to Expect

- After the infection is gone, the nodes slowly return to normal size.
- This may take 2 to 4 weeks.
- However, they won't ever completely go away.

❽ Call Your Doctor If

- Node grows 1 in (2.5 cm) or larger in size.
- Big node lasts more than 1 month.
- You think your child needs to be seen.
- Your child becomes worse.

Remember!
Contact your doctor if your child develops any of the **Call Your Doctor** symptoms.

CHAPTER 22

Mouth Ulcers

Definition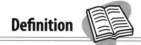

▶ Painful, shallow ulcers (sores) on the lining of the mouth.

▶ Sores found on the gums, inner lips, inner cheeks, or tongue.

▶ Sores only on the outer lips (such as cold sores).

Causes of Mouth Ulcers or Sores

▶ **Canker sores.** The main cause of 1 or 2 mouth ulcers after age 5.

▶ **Hand-foot-and-mouth disease.** The most common cause of multiple ulcers in the mouth. These ulcers are mainly on the tongue and sides of the mouth. Most children also have small, deep blisters on the palms and soles. This is due to the Coxsackie virus. It is common between ages 1 to 5 years.

▶ **Herpes gingivostomatitis.** The first infection with the herpes cold sore virus can be severe. It can cause 10 or more ulcers on the gums, tongue, and inner lips. Ulcers also occur on the outer lips and skin around the mouth. Ulcers are present on both sides of the mouth. Fever, pain, and trouble swallowing are present. Usually occurs between ages 1 to 3. May follow contact with an older child or adult who has active cold sores (fever blisters). Often after the infected person has kissed the child.

▶ **Recurrent cold sores (fever blisters).** Sores are found on the outer lip and only on one side. They recur several times a year, always in the same place. No ulcers are found inside the mouth. Recurrent fever blisters occur in 20% of teens and adults.

▶ **Mouth injury.** Common mouth injuries are biting the tongue or inside of the cheek. Others can be caused by a toothbrush. The lining of the mouth always looks white when it heals. Forgotten injuries can look like a canker sore.

▶ **Mouth burns.** Hot foods (such as pizza) can cause mouth sores. They also turn white as they heal.

Causes of Canker Sores

▶ Canker sores have many causes.

▶ Minor injuries to the mouth can trigger a canker sore. Examples are from a rough food or hard toothbrush. Biting oneself while chewing can start one.

- Food allergies or irritants may also be a trigger.

- Vitamin deficiencies can also be a cause. A vitamin deficiency can occur if your child is a picky eater.

- Canker sores can run in families (genetic).

- Often, the cause is unknown.

Symptoms of Canker Sores

- Small ulcers have a white center with a red border around them.

- Size is usually less than ¼ in or 6 mm.

- Found on the inner lips and inner cheeks.

- The sores are very painful, even when not eating.

- Usually 1 canker sore develops at a time. Sometimes 2 or 3 develop.

- No fever or other symptoms.

When to Call Your Doctor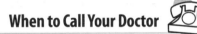

Call 911 Now (Your Child May Need an Ambulance) If

- Not moving or too weak to stand.

- You think your child has a life-threatening emergency.

Call Your Doctor Now (Night or Day) If

- Chemical in the mouth could have caused ulcers.

- Dehydration suspected (no urine in more than 8 hours, dark urine, very dry mouth, and no tears).

- Your child looks or acts very sick.

- You think your child needs to be seen, and the problem is urgent.

Call Your Doctor Within 24 Hours If

- Four or more ulcers.

- Bloody crusts on the lips.

- Red, swollen, tender gums.

- Ulcers and sores also on the outer lips.

- One ulcer on the gum near a tooth with a toothache.

► Fever or swollen face.

► Large lymph node under the jaw.

► Began after starting a medicine.

► You think your child needs to be seen, but the problem is not urgent.

Call Your Doctor During Weekday Office Hours If

► Cold sores are suspected.

► Mouth ulcers last more than 2 weeks.

► You have other questions or concerns.

Parent Care at Home If

► Canker sores suspected.

Care Advice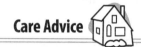

❶ What You Should Know About Mouth Ulcers

■ Canker sores are the most common cause of mouth ulcers.

■ They are 1 to 3 painful, white ulcers of the inner cheeks, inner lip, or gums (no fever).

■ Causes include injuries from rough food, toothbrushes, biting, or food irritants.

■ Here is some care advice that should help.

❷ Liquid Antacid for Mouth Pain (Age: 1 Year and Older)

■ For mouth pain, use a liquid antacid (such as Mylanta or the store brand). Give 4 times per day as needed. After meals is often a good time.

■ **Age:** 1 to 6 years. Put a few drops in the mouth. Can also put it on with a cotton swab.

■ **Age:** Older than 6 years. Use 1 teaspoon (5 mL) as a mouthwash. Keep it on the ulcers as long as possible. Then spit it out. It is safe to swallow it.

■ Can use honey instead until you can buy a liquid antacid. Follow the same directions as given for antacids. Avoid honey if younger than 1 year.

■ **Caution:** Do not use regular mouthwashes, because they sting.

❸ Pain Medicine

- To help with pain, give an acetaminophen product (such as Tylenol).
- Another choice is an ibuprofen product (such as Advil).
- Use as needed.

❹ Fluids and Soft Diet

- Try to get your child to drink adequate fluids.
- **Goal:** Keep your child well hydrated.
- Cold drinks, milk shakes, Popsicles, slushes, and sherbet are good choices.
- Solid foods: Soft, bland foods such as macaroni and cheese. Other options include mashed potatoes, cereals with milk, and ice cream.
- Avoid foods that need much chewing. Avoid citrus, salty, or spicy foods. (Note: Fluid intake is more important than eating any solids.)
- For infants, you may need to stop the bottle. Give fluids by cup, spoon, or syringe instead. (**Reason:** The nipple can increase the pain.)

❺ Return to School

- Canker sores cannot be spread to others. Children with canker sores do not need to miss any school.
- Children with fever need to be checked before going back to school.
- Also, children with many mouth ulcers should be checked before going back.

❻ What to Expect

- They heal in 1 to 2 weeks on their own.
- Once they occur, no treatment can shorten the illness.
- Treatment can help with the pain.

❼ Call Your Doctor If

- Mouth ulcers last more than 2 weeks.
- You think your child needs to be seen.
- Your child becomes worse.

Remember!
Contact your doctor if your child develops any of the **Call Your Doctor** symptoms.

CHAPTER 23

Mouth Injury

Definition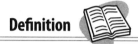

- ▶ Injuries to the lips and mouth.
- ▶ Includes inner cheeks and roof of the mouth (hard and soft palate).
- ▶ Front of the mouth includes the tongue. Also, includes the flap under the upper lip (frenulum).
- ▶ Back of the mouth includes the tonsils and the throat.

See Other Chapter If
- ▶ Main injury is to teeth. See Chapter 24, Tooth Injury.

Types of Mouth Injuries
- ▶ **Tongue.** Cuts on the tongue or inside the cheeks are the most common mouth injury. Usually, these are due to unintentionally biting them during eating. Bites of the tongue rarely need sutures. Even if they gape open a little, the cuts usually heal quickly. If the edges come together when the tongue is still, it needs no treatment.
- ▶ **Upper lip.** Cuts and bruises of the upper lip are usually due to falls. The piece of tissue joining the upper lip to the gum is the frenulum. A tear of the upper frenulum is very common. It always heals without sutures. However, it will rebleed every time you pull the lip out to look at it. Gaping cut of the lip or through lip border may need stitches.
- ▶ **Lower lip.** Cuts of the lower lip are usually caused by the teeth. They occur when catching the lip between the upper and lower teeth while falling. Most of these cuts do not connect (don't go through the lip). These do not need sutures unless the outer cut is gaping.
- ▶ Serious injuries are those to the tonsils, soft palate, or back of the throat. Examples of these injuries include falling with a pencil or toothbrush in the mouth. Puncture wounds here can cause a deep space infection in the neck.

When to Call Your Doctor

Call 911 Now (Your Child May Need an Ambulance) If

- Major bleeding that can't be stopped.
- Trouble breathing.
- You think your child has a life-threatening emergency.

Go to ER Now If

- Minor bleeding (more than oozing) won't stop after 10 minutes of direct pressure.
- Injury to back of the mouth caused by a long object (such as a pencil).
- Large, deep cut that will need many stitches.

Call Your Doctor Now (Night or Day) If

- Gaping cut on the tongue or inside the mouth may need stitches.
- Gaping cut of the lip may need stitches.
- Severe pain has not improved 2 hours after taking pain medicine.
- Trouble swallowing fluids or saliva.
- Can't fully open or close the mouth.
- Fever present and mouth looks infected. Signs are increasing pain or swelling after 48 hours. (**Note:** It's normal for a healing wound in the mouth to be white.)
- You think your child has a serious injury.
- You think your child needs to be seen, and the problem is urgent.

Call Your Doctor Within 24 Hours If

- Mouth looks infected and no fever is present.
- You think your child needs to be seen, but the problem is not urgent.

Call Your Doctor During Weekday Office Hours If

- You have other questions or concerns.

Parent Care at Home If

- Minor mouth injury.

Care Advice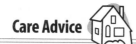

❶ Upper Lip and Frenulum Bleeding: How to Stop It

- Cuts on the inside, upper lip are very common.
- Often, the piece of tissue that connects the upper lip to the upper gum is torn. This tissue is called the *upper labial frenulum.*
- The main symptom is oozing tiny amounts of blood.
- This cut always heals perfectly without sutures.
- For bleeding from the frenulum, use direct pressure. Press the outer lip against the teeth for 10 minutes.
- **Caution:** Once bleeding has stopped, don't pull the lip out to look at it. (**Reason:** Bleeding will start up again.)
- It's safe to check it after 3 days.

❷ Lower Lip Bleeding: How to Stop It

- Most children who fall and bite their lower lip have 2 cuts. They have cuts to both the outside and inside of the lip.
- Catching the lower lip between the upper and lower teeth causes the 2 cuts. This tends to happen in children with an overbite.
- Most of these small cuts do not connect with each other.
- For bleeding from the lip, use direct pressure. Press the outer lip against the teeth for 10 minutes.

❸ Tongue Bleeding: How to Stop It

- Bites of the tongue rarely need sutures.
- Even if they gape open a little, tongue cuts usually heal quickly. If the edges come together when the tongue is still, it needs no treatment.
- For tongue bleeding, try to press on the bleeding site with a sterile gauze. You can also use a piece of clean cloth. Do this for 5 minutes if it's practical.
- Cuts of the tongue normally tend to ooze a little blood for several hours. This is due to the rich blood supply in the mouth.
- For constant oozing of blood, can use a moistened tea bag for 10 minutes. (**Reason:** Tannic acid released from the tea bag may stop the oozing.)

❹ Cold for Pain

- Put a piece of ice or Popsicle on the spot that was injured.
- You can also use a cold, wet washcloth.
- Do this for 20 minutes.

❺ Pain Medicine

- To help with pain, give an acetaminophen product (such as Tylenol).
- Another choice is an ibuprofen product (such as Advil).
- Use as needed.

❻ Soft Diet

- Try to get your child to drink adequate fluids.
- **Goal:** Keep your child well hydrated.
- Cold drinks, milk shakes, Popsicles, slushes, and sherbet are good choices.
- Solids: Offer a soft diet. Also, avoid foods that need much chewing. Avoid citrus, salty, or spicy foods.
- Rinse the wound with warm water right after meals.

❼ What to Expect

- Small cuts and scrapes inside the mouth heal in 3 or 4 days.
- Infections of mouth injuries are rare.

❽ Call Your Doctor If

- Pain becomes severe.
- Mouth looks infected (mainly, increasing pain or swelling after 48 hours).
- Fever occurs.
- You think your child needs to be seen.
- Your child becomes worse.

Remember!
Contact your doctor if your child develops any of the **Call Your Doctor** symptoms.

CHAPTER 24

Tooth Injury

Definition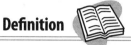

▶ Injury to a tooth.

Types of Tooth Injuries

▶ **Loosened tooth.** May bleed a little from the gums. Usually tightens up on its own.

▶ **Displaced tooth.** Usually pushed inward. Needs to be seen.

▶ **Chipped tooth.** Minor fracture with small corner of tooth missing. The fracture goes to the dentin (yellow color), not the pulp (red color). Not painful. See dentist during office hours.

▶ **Fractured tooth.** The fracture goes down to the pulp. The pulp is where the blood supply and nerves to the tooth are located. The main finding is a red dot or bleeding in the center of the tooth. Very painful. Needs a root canal to save the tooth.

▶ **Knocked-out permanent tooth.** Also called an *avulsed tooth*. A dental emergency. Needs to be reimplanted within 2 hours.

▶ **Knocked-out baby tooth.** It cannot be reimplanted. See dentist during office hours.

Symptoms

▶ The main symptom is pain.

▶ Minor bleeding from the gums may occur.

First Aid for Knocked-Out Permanent Tooth (Not for Baby Teeth)

▶ To save the tooth, it must be put back in as soon as possible. Two hours is the outer limit for survival. Right away is best. If more than 30 minutes away from dental care, try to replace the tooth. Put it back in the socket before coming in. Use the method below.

• Rinse off the tooth with saliva or water (do not scrub it).

• Replace it in the socket facing the correct way.

- Press down on the tooth with your thumb. Do this until the crown is level with the tooth next to it.

- Have your teen bite down on a wad of cloth. This will help to stabilize the tooth until you can reach your dentist.

- Putting a tooth back in the socket can be difficult because of pain and bleeding. If unsuccessful for 10 minutes, take the tooth with you to the dentist or ER.

- **Note:** Baby teeth can't be reimplanted. (Give them to the tooth fairy!)

Transporting a Knocked-Out Permanent Tooth

▸ If not able to put the tooth back in its socket, follow these instructions.

- It is very important to keep the tooth moist. Do not let it dry out.

- Transport the tooth in cow's milk or saliva. Milk is best per the American Dental Association (2003).

- **Milk transport option 1 (best):** Place the tooth in a small plastic bag with some milk. Put the plastic bag in a cup of ice.

- **Milk transport option 2:** Place the tooth in a cup of cold milk.

- **Saliva transport option 1:** Put the tooth inside your child's mouth. Your child should be careful not to swallow it. (**Exception:** Child who is younger than 12 years.)

- **Saliva transport option 2:** Put the tooth in a cup. Keep the tooth moist with your child's saliva (spit).

When to Call Your Doctor

Go to ER Now If

▸ Bleeding won't stop after 10 minutes of direct pressure.

Call Your Dentist or Doctor Now (Night or Day) If

▸ Permanent (adult) tooth knocked out. (**Reason:** Needs to be put back within 2 hours to survive.)

▸ Permanent (adult) tooth is almost falling out.

▸ Baby tooth is almost falling out after injury.

▸ Tooth is greatly pushed out of its normal place.

- Tooth that's pushed out of its normal place makes it hard to chew.
- Severe pain has not improved 2 hours after taking pain medicine.
- **Age:** Younger than 1 year.
- You think your child has a serious injury.
- You think your child needs to be seen, and the problem is urgent.

Call Your Dentist Within 24 Hours If

- You think your child needs to be seen, but the problem is not urgent.
- Baby tooth knocked out by injury. (**Reason:** Can't be put back. However, a dentist does need to check for damage to the permanent tooth inside the gum.)
- Tooth is slightly pushed out of its normal place.
- Chip or crack in the tooth.
- Tooth feels very loose when you try to move it.

Call Your Dentist During Weekday Office Hours If

- Cold fluids cause tooth pain.
- Tooth turns a darker color.
- Crown or cap comes off. (**Note:** Save the crown for the dentist.)
- You have other questions or concerns.

Parent Care at Home If

- Minor tooth injury.

Care Advice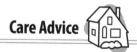

❶ Cold for Pain

- For pain, place a piece of ice or a Popsicle on the injured gum.
- You can also use a cold pack on the cheek.
- Apply for 20 minutes.

❷ Pain Medicine

- To help with pain, give an acetaminophen product (such as Tylenol).
- Another choice is an ibuprofen product (such as Advil).
- Use as needed.

❸ Soft Diet

- For any loose teeth, offer a soft diet.

- Avoid foods that need a lot of chewing.

- You can go back to a normal diet after 3 days. By then, the tooth should be tightened up.

❹ What to Expect

- Tooth pain most often goes away in 2 or 3 days.

❺ Call Your Dentist If

- Pain becomes severe.

- Cold fluids cause tooth pain.

- Tooth turns a darker color.

- You think your child needs to be seen.

- Your child becomes worse.

Remember!
Contact your doctor if your child develops any of the **Call Your Doctor** symptoms.

PART 7

Lung or Breathing Symptoms

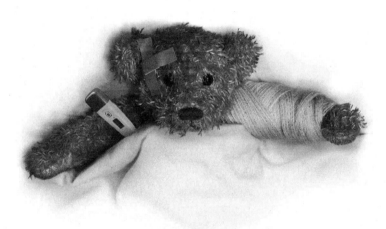

CHAPTER 25

Asthma Attack

Definition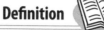

▶ Your child is having an asthma attack.

▶ Use this chapter only if a doctor has told you your child has asthma.

Symptoms of Asthma Attack

▶ Symptoms of an asthma attack are wheezing, a cough, tight chest, and trouble breathing.

▶ Wheezing is the classic symptom. Wheezing is a high-pitched whistling or purring sound. You can hear it best when your child is breathing out.

▶ Diagnosis of asthma requires attacks of wheezing that recur. The diagnosis is rarely made before 1 year of age.

Causes (Triggers) of Asthma Attacks

▶ **Infections** that affect breathing (like colds or the flu).

▶ **Pollens** (trees, grass, and weeds).

▶ **Animals** (like cats or rabbits).

▶ **Tobacco smoke.**

▶ **Irritants** (such as smog, car exhaust, menthol vapors, barns, or a dirty basement).

▶ **Food allergy (serious).** Asthma attacks caused by food allergy can be life-threatening (lead to anaphylaxis). Examples are nuts or fish.

Asthma Attack Scale

▶ **Peak flow meter:** A peak flow meter measures peak flow rates. It tells us how well a person can move air out of the lungs. It can be used in children 6 years and older.

▶ **Mild:** No shortness of breath (SOB) at rest. Mild SOB with walking. Can talk normally. Speaks in sentences. Can lie down flat. Wheezes not heard or mild. (**Green zone:** Peak flow rate is 80%–100% of normal rate.)

▸ **Moderate:** SOB at rest. Speaks in phrases. Wants to sit (can't lie down flat). Wheezing can be heard. Retractions are present (ribs pull in with each breath). (**Yellow zone:** Peak flow rate is 50%–80% of normal rate.)

▸ **Severe:** Severe SOB at rest. Speaks in single words. Struggling to breathe. Wheezing may be loud. Rarely, wheezing is absent because of poor air movement. Retractions may be severe. (**Red zone:** Peak flow rate is less than 50% of normal rate.)

First Aid for Anaphylaxis: Epinephrine

▸ Anaphylaxis is a life-threatening allergic reaction.

▸ If you have epinephrine (such as EpiPen or Auvi-Q), give it now.

▸ Do this while calling 911.

▸ Above 66 lb (30 kg): Give 0.3 mg EpiPen.

▸ Between 22 and 66 lb (10–30 kg): Give 0.15 mg EpiPen Jr.

▸ Less than 22 lb (10 kg): Give dose advised by your doctor.

▸ Give the shot into the upper, outer thigh in the leg straight down.

▸ Can be given through clothing if needed.

▸ A second shot should be given if no improvement in 10 minutes.

▸ **Albuterol inhaler:** After giving the EpiPen, give 4 puffs from your child's asthma inhaler.

▸ Benadryl: After giving the EpiPen, also give Benadryl by mouth. Do this if your child is able to swallow.

When to Call Your Doctor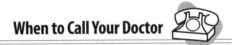

Call 911 Now (Your Child May Need an Ambulance) If

▸ Wheezing and life-threatening allergic reaction to similar substance in the past.

▸ Starts to wheeze suddenly after bee sting, taking a new medicine, or allergic food.

▸ Severe trouble breathing (struggling for each breath, can barely speak or cry).

▸ Passed out.

▸ Lips or face are bluish when not coughing.

▸ You think your child has a life-threatening emergency.

Go to ER Now If

▶ Looks like he did when hospitalized before with asthma.

▶ Trouble breathing not gone 20 minutes after nebulizer or inhaler.

▶ Peak flow rate is less than 50% of normal rate (red zone).

▶ Ribs are pulling in with each breath (retractions).

Call Your Doctor Now (Night or Day) If

▶ Pulse oxygen level is less than 90% during asthma attack.

▶ Lips or face have turned bluish during coughing.

▶ Peak flow rate is 50% to 80% of normal rate after using nebulizer or inhaler (yellow zone).

▶ Wheezing not gone 20 minutes after using nebulizer or inhaler.

▶ Breathing much faster than normal.

▶ Nonstop coughing has not improved after using nebulizer or inhaler.

▶ Severe chest pain.

▶ Need to use asthma medicine (nebulizer or inhaler) more often than every 4 hours.

▶ Fever above 104°F (40°C).

▶ Your child looks or acts very sick.

▶ You think your child needs to be seen, and the problem is urgent.

Call Your Doctor Within 24 Hours If

▶ Mild wheezing lasts more than 24 hours on nebulizer or inhaler treatments.

▶ Sinus pain (not just congestion).

▶ Fever lasts more than 3 days.

▶ Fever returns after being gone for more than 24 hours.

▶ You think your child needs to be seen, but the problem is not urgent.

Call Your Doctor During Weekday Office Hours If

▶ You don't have written asthma action plan from your doctor.

▶ Your child uses an inhaler but doesn't have a spacer.

▶ Misses more than 1 day of school per month for asthma.

▶ Asthma limits exercise or sports.

▶ Asthma attacks wake your child up from sleep.

▶ Uses more than 1 inhaler per month.

▶ No asthma checkup in more than 1 year.

▶ You have other questions or concerns.

Parent Care at Home If

▶ Mild asthma attack.

Care Advice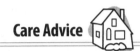

❶ What You Should Know About Asthma

■ More than 10% of children have asthma.

■ Your child's asthma can flare up at any time.

■ When you are away from your home, always take your child's medicines with you.

■ The sooner you start treatment, the faster your child will feel better.

■ Here is some care advice that should help.

❷ Asthma Quick-Relief Medicine

■ Your child's quick-relief (rescue) medicine is albuterol or Xopenex.

■ Start it at the first sign of any wheezing, shortness of breath, or hard coughing.

■ Give by inhaler with a spacer (2 puffs each time) or use a nebulizer machine.

■ Repeat it every 4 hours if your child is having any asthma symptoms.

■ Never give it more often than every 4 hours without talking with your child's doctor.

■ **Coughing.** The best "cough medicine" for a child with asthma is always the asthma medicine. (**Caution:** Don't use cough suppressants. For older than 6 years, cough drops may help a tickly cough.)

■ **Caution:** If the inhaler hasn't been used in more than 7 days, prime it. Test spray it twice into the air before using it for treatment. Also, do this if it is new.

■ Use the medicine until your child has not wheezed or coughed for 48 hours.

■ **Spacer.** Always use inhalers with a spacer. It will get twice the amount of medicine into the lungs.

❸ Asthma Controller Medicine

- Your child may have been told to use a controller drug. An example is an inhaled steroid.
- It's for preventing attacks and must be used daily.
- During asthma attacks, keep giving this medicine to your child as ordered.

❹ Allergy Medicine for Hay Fever

- For signs of nasal allergies (hay fever), it's OK to give allergy medicine. (**Reason:** Poor control of nasal allergies makes asthma worse.)

❺ Fluids: Offer More

- Try to get your child to drink lots of fluids.
- **Goal:** Keep your child well hydrated.
- **Reason:** It will loosen up any phlegm in the lungs. Then it's easier to cough up.

❻ Humidifier

- If the air in your home is dry, use a humidifier. (**Reason:** Dry air makes coughs worse.)

❼ Avoid Tobacco Smoke

- Tobacco smoke makes asthma much worse.
- Don't let anyone smoke around your child.

❽ Avoid or Remove Triggers

- Shower to remove pollens or other allergens from the body and hair.
- Avoid known causes of asthma attacks (such as smoke or cats).
- During attacks, reduce exercise or sports if it makes the asthma worse.

❾ What to Expect

- If treatment is started early, most asthma attacks are quickly brought under control.
- All wheezing should be gone within 5 days.

❿ Inhaler With a Spacer: How to Use It

- **Step 1.** Shake the inhaler well. Then attach it to the spacer (holding chamber).
- **Step 2.** Have your child breathe out completely and empty the lungs.

- **Step 3.** Place the mouthpiece of the spacer in the mouth.

- **Step 4.** Press down on the inhaler. This will put one puff of the medicine in the spacer.

- **Step 5.** Have your child breathe in slowly for 5 seconds until the lungs are full.

- **Step 6.** Ask your child to hold a deep breath for 10 seconds. Allow the medicine to work deep in the lungs.

- **Note:** If your doctor has ordered 2 or more puffs, wait 1 minute. Then repeat steps 2 to 6.

⑪ Metered Dose Inhaler: How to Use It Without a Spacer

- **Step 1.** Shake the inhaler well.

- **Step 2.** Breathe out completely and empty the lungs.

- **Step 3.** Close the lips and teeth around the inhaler mouthpiece.

- **Step 4.** Press down on the inhaler to release a puff. Do this just as your child starts to breathe in.

- **Step 5.** Have your child breathe in slowly until the lungs are full.

- **Step 6.** Ask your child to hold a deep breath for 10 seconds. Allow the medicine to work deep in the lungs.

- **Note:** If your doctor has ordered 2 or more puffs, wait 1 minute. Then repeat steps 1 to 6.

- **Spacer.** Ask your doctor for a spacer if you don't have one. It will help send more medicine into the lungs.

- Older children who don't like a spacer can be prescribed an albuterol dry powder device.

⑫ Home Nebulizer: How to Use It

- A nebulizer machine changes a liquid medicine into a fine mist. The fine mist can carry the medicine deep into the lungs. This is called *a nebulizer treatment.*

  - **Step 1.** Prepare the medicine. First, wash your hands with soap and water. For premixed single dose vials, just add one vial to the nebulizer holding cup. For multidose vials, you need to do the mixing. First, add the correct amount of normal saline solution to the nebulizer cup. Then carefully measure and add the correct amount of medicine to the saline.

- **Step 2.** Connect the nebulizer to the air compressor tubing. The air compressor is run by electricity. Portable ones run on a battery. Compressors make the jet of air that turns the medicine into a fine mist.

- **Step 3.** Turn on the air compressor. It will start making the fine mist that your child needs.

- **Step 4 for an *older child*.** Place the mouthpiece between your child's teeth and have him seal it with the lips. Ask your child to breathe slowly and deeply. Ask your child to hold a deep breath for 10 seconds once a minute.

- **Step 4 for a *younger child*.** If your child refuses the mouthpiece, use a face mask. It should cover the nose and mouth. It should fit snugly.

- **Step 5.** Continue treatment until the medicine is gone. If the medicine sticks to the side of the cup, shake it a little. An average nebulizer treatment takes 10 minutes.

- **Step 6.** After each treatment, take the nebulizer apart. Rinse and clean it as directed. (**Reason:** It can't produce mist if it becomes clogged up.)

■ **Caution:** Closely follow your doctor's instructions. Use the exact amount of medicine your doctor ordered. Don't give a nebulizer treatment more often than every 4 hours.

⓭ Call Your Doctor If

■ Trouble breathing occurs.

■ Asthma quick-relief medicine (nebulizer or inhaler) is needed more than every 4 hours.

■ Wheezing lasts more than 24 hours.

■ You think your child needs to be seen.

■ Your child becomes worse.

Remember!
Contact your doctor if your child develops any of the **Call Your Doctor** symptoms.

CHAPTER 26

Cough

Definition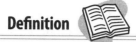

- The sound made when the cough reflex clears the airway of irritants.
- Most coughs are part of a cold.
- A coughing fit or spell is more than 5 minutes of nonstop coughing.

See Other Chapter If

- Stridor (harsh sound with breathing in), barky cough, or hoarse voice. See Chapter 27, Croup.
- Your child has asthma. See Chapter 25, Asthma Attack.

Causes of Cough

- **Common cold.** Most coughs are part of a cold that includes the lower airway. The medical name is *viral bronchitis*. Bronchi are the lower part of the airway that goes to the lungs. Bronchitis in children is always caused by a virus. This includes cold viruses, influenza, and croup. Bacteria do not cause bronchitis in healthy children.
- **Sinus infection.** The exact mechanism of the cough is unknown. It may be that postnasal drip irritates the lower throat or pressure within the sinus may trigger the cough reflex.
- **Allergic cough.** Some children get a cough from breathing in an allergic substance. Examples are pollens or cat dander. Allergic coughs can be controlled with allergy medicines, such as Benadryl.
- **Asthma.** Asthma with wheezing is the most common cause of chronic coughs in children. In adults, it's smoking.
- **Cough-variant asthma.** 25% of children with asthma only cough and never wheeze. The coughing spells have the same triggers as asthma attacks.
- **Air pollution cough.** Fumes of any kind can irritate the airway and cause a cough. Tobacco smoke is the most common example. Others are automobile exhaust, smog, and paint fumes.

▸ **Exercise-induced cough.** Running will make most coughs worse. If the air is cold or polluted, coughing is even more likely.

▸ **Serious causes.** Pneumonia, bronchiolitis, whooping cough, and foreign body (object) in the airway.

Trouble Breathing: How to Tell It's Happening

▸ Trouble breathing is a reason to see a doctor right away. *Respiratory distress* is the medical name for trouble breathing. Here are symptoms to worry about.

- Struggling for each breath or shortness of breath.

- Breathing is so tight that your child can barely speak or cry.

- Ribs are pulling in with each breath (called *retractions*).

- Breathing has become noisy (such as wheezes).

- Breathing is much faster than normal.

- Lips or face turn a blue color.

Phlegm or Sputum: What's Normal?

▸ Yellow or green phlegm is a normal part of healing from viral bronchitis.

▸ This means lining of the trachea (windpipe) was damaged by the virus. It's part of the phlegm your child coughs up.

▸ Bacteria do not cause bronchitis in healthy children. Antibiotics are not helpful for the yellow or green phlegm seen with colds.

▸ The main treatment of a cough with phlegm is to drink lots of fluids. Also, if the air is dry, using a humidifier will help. Sipping warm clear fluids will also help coughing fits.

Vaping Risk

▸ Talk with your child about the dangers of vaping.

▸ Vaping can cause severe lung injury. The lung damage can be permanent.

▸ Vaping can even cause death.

▸ Vaping tobacco also causes nicotine addiction.

▸ The legal age to purchase vaping products is 21 years in the United States.

▸ Encourage your teen to avoid vaping. If they have started, urge them to quit.

▸ **Warning:** Never use homemade or street-purchased vaping solutions. (**Reason:** They have caused the most lung damage.)

When to Call Your Doctor

Call 911 Now (Your Child May Need an Ambulance) If

- Severe trouble breathing (struggling for each breath, can barely speak or cry).
- Passed out or stopped breathing.
- Lips or face are bluish when not coughing.
- You think your child has a life-threatening emergency.

Go to ER Now If

- Choked on a small object that could be caught in the throat.
- Ribs are pulling in with each breath (retractions).
- Not alert when awake (out of it).

Call Your Doctor Now (Night or Day) If

- Trouble breathing, but not severe.
- Lips or face have turned bluish during coughing.
- Harsh sound with breathing in (called *stridor*).
- Wheezing (purring or whistling sound during breathing out).
- Breathing is much faster than normal.
- Can't take a deep breath because of chest pain.
- Severe chest pain.
- Coughed up blood.
- Weak immune system (such as sickle cell disease, HIV, cancer, organ transplant, or taking oral steroids).
- High-risk child (such as with cystic fibrosis or other chronic lung disease).
- **Age:** Younger than 12 weeks with fever. (**Caution:** Do *not* give your baby any fever medicine before being seen.)
- Fever above 104°F (40°C).
- Your child looks or acts very sick.
- You think your child needs to be seen, and the problem is urgent.

Call Your Doctor Within 24 Hours If

▶ Nonstop coughing spells.

▶ **Age:** Younger than 6 months.

▶ Earache or ear discharge.

▶ Sinus pain (not just congestion) around cheekbone or eyes.

▶ Fever lasts more than 3 days.

▶ Fever returns after being gone for more than 24 hours.

▶ Chest pain, even when not coughing.

▶ Concerns about vaping.

▶ You think your child needs to be seen, but the problem is not urgent.

Call Your Doctor During Weekday Office Hours If

▶ Coughing causes vomiting 3 or more times.

▶ Coughing has kept your child home from school for 3 or more days.

▶ Allergic symptoms (such as runny nose and itchy eyes) also present.

▶ Runny nose lasts more than 14 days.

▶ Cough lasts more than 3 weeks.

▶ You have other questions or concerns.

Parent Care at Home If

▶ Cough with no complications.

Care Advice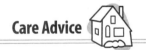

❶ What You Should Know About Coughs

■ Most coughs are a normal part of a cold.

■ Coughing up mucus is very important. It helps protect the lungs from pneumonia.

■ A cough can be a good thing. We don't want to fully turn off a child's ability to cough.

■ Here is some care advice that should help.

❷ Homemade Cough Medicine

- Coughing has a purpose. It protects the lungs. It does not need any treatment. Just keep your child well hydrated. (**Reason:** A dry throat and airway increases the coughing.) If you wish, you can also try warm fluids for bad coughing.

- **Age:** Younger than 6 months: Only give breast milk or formula.

- **Age:** 6 to 12 months. Try an ounce (30 mL) of warm water or apple juice. **Caution:** Do not use honey until 1 year of age.

- **Age:** 1 year and older. Honey is the best choice. Give ½ to 1 teaspoon (2.5–5 mL) as needed. It can thin secretions and soothe the throat. If you don't have any honey, you can use corn syrup. Can also offer warm fruit juice, herbal teas, or other clear fluid. **Amount:** A few ounces (30 mL) each time.

- **Age:** 6 years and older. Use cough drops to decrease any tickle in the throat. If you don't have any, you can use hard candy. Honey can also help. **Caution:** Avoid cough drops before 6 years. (**Reason:** Risk of choking.)

❸ Nonprescription Cough Medicine

- Nonprescription cough medicines are not advised. (**Reason:** No proven benefit for children and not approved by the US Food and Drug Administration for children younger than 6 years.)

- Honey has been shown to work better for coughs. (**Caution:** Do not use honey until 1 year of age.)

- Cough drops are a good choice after age 6.

❹ Coughing Fits or Spells: Warm Mist and Fluids

- Breathe warm mist (such as from a shower running in a closed bathroom).

- Also give warm clear fluids to drink. **Age:** Must be older than 6 months.

- **Age:** 6 to 12 months. Warm water often helps.

- **Age:** 1 year and older. Use any warm clear fluid your child likes, such as fruit juice, flavored water, or herbal teas.

- **Reason:** Warm mist and warm fluids both relax the airway and loosen up any phlegm.

❺ Vomiting From Hard Coughing

- For vomiting that occurs with hard coughing, give smaller amounts per feeding.

- Also, feed more often.

- **Reason:** Vomiting from coughing is more common with a full stomach.

➏ Encourage Fluids

- Try to get your child to drink lots of fluids.
- **Goal:** Keep your child well hydrated.
- It also loosens up any phlegm in the lungs. Then it's easier to cough up.
- It will also thin out mucus discharge from the nose.

➐ Humidifier

- If the air in your home is dry, use a humidifier. (**Reason:** Dry air makes coughs worse.)

➑ Fever Medicine

- For fevers above 102°F (39°C), give an acetaminophen product (such as Tylenol).
- Another choice is an ibuprofen product (such as Advil).
- **Note:** Fevers under 102°F (39°C) are important for fighting infections.
- **For all fevers:** Keep your child well hydrated. Give lots of cold fluids.

➒ Avoid Tobacco Smoke

- Tobacco smoke makes coughs much worse.

➓ Return to School

- Your child can go back to school after the fever is gone.
- Your child should also feel well enough to join in normal activities.
- For practical purposes, the spread of coughs and colds cannot be prevented.

⓫ Extra Advice: Allergy Medicine for Allergic Cough

- Allergy medicine can bring an allergic cough under control within 1 hour. The same is true for nasal allergic symptoms.
- A short-acting allergy medicine (such as Benadryl) is helpful. No prescription is needed.
- Do not use Benadryl longer than a few days. Age limit: 1 year and older.
- Switch to a long-acting antihistamine after a few days, such as Zyrtec. Age limit: 2 years and older.

⑫ What to Expect

- Viral coughs most often last for 2 to 3 weeks.

- Sometimes, your child will cough up lots of phlegm (mucus). Mucus is normally gray, yellow, or green.

- Antibiotics are not helpful.

⑬ Call Your Doctor If

- Trouble breathing occurs.

- Wheezing occurs.

- Cough lasts more than 3 weeks.

- You think your child needs to be seen.

- Your child becomes worse.

Remember!
Contact your doctor if your child develops any of the **Call Your Doctor** symptoms.

CHAPTER 27

Croup

Definition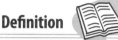

- ► Barky cough and hoarse voice caused by a virus.
- ► Croup is a viral infection of the voice box (larynx).
- ► Croupy cough is tight, low-pitched, and barky (like a barking seal).
- ► The voice or cry is hoarse (called *laryngitis*).
- ► Some children with severe croup get a harsh, tight sound while breathing in. This is called *stridor*.

See Other Chapter If

- ► It doesn't sound like croup. See Chapter 26, Cough.

Stridor: A Complication of Croup

- ► Stridor is a harsh, raspy tight sound best heard with breathing in.
- ► Loud or constant stridor means severe croup. Stridor at rest (when not crying or coughing) also means severe croup.
- ► All stridor needs to be treated with warm mist.
- ► Most children with stridor need treatment with a steroid (such as Decadron).
- ► For any stridor, see this chapter's Care Advice or First Aid for Stridor section for treatment.

Causes of a Croupy Cough

- ► **Viral croup.** Viruses are the most common cause of croup symptoms. Many respiratory viruses can infect the vocal cord area and cause narrowing. Even influenza (the flu) can do this. A fever is often present with barky cough.
- ► **Allergic croup.** A croupy cough can occur with exposure to pollens or allergens. A runny nose, itchy eyes, and sneezing are also often present.

- ▶ **Inhaled powder.** Breathing in any fine substance can trigger 10 minutes of severe coughing. Examples are powdered sugar, flour dust, or peanut dust. They can float into the lungs. This is not an allergic reaction.

- ▶ **Foreign body in the airway (serious).** Suspect this when there is a sudden onset of coughing and choking. Common examples are peanut and seeds. Peak age is 1 to 4 years.

- ▶ **Food allergy (serious).** Croup symptoms can also be caused by a food allergy. This can be life-threatening (lead to anaphylaxis). Examples are nuts or fish.

First Aid for Stridor (Harsh Sound With Breathing In) or Nonstop Coughing

- ▶ Breathe warm mist in a closed bathroom with the hot shower running. Do this for 20 minutes.

- ▶ You could also use a wet washcloth held near the face.

- ▶ **Caution:** Do not use very hot water or steam, which could cause burns.

- ▶ If warm mist fails, breathe cool air by standing near an open refrigerator. You can also go outside with your child if the weather is cold. Do this for a few minutes.

When to Call Your Doctor

Call 911 Now (Your Child May Need an Ambulance) If

- ▶ Severe trouble breathing (struggling for each breath, constant severe stridor).

- ▶ Passed out or stopped breathing.

- ▶ Lips or face are bluish when not coughing.

- ▶ Croup started suddenly after bee sting, taking a new medicine, or exposure to an allergic food.

- ▶ Drooling, spitting, or having great trouble swallowing. (**Exception:** Drooling due to teething.)

- ▶ You think your child has a life-threatening emergency.

Go to ER Now If

- ▶ Choked on a small object that could be caught in the throat.

- ▶ Ribs are pulling in with each breath (retractions).

- ▶ **Age:** Younger than 1 year with stridor (harsh sound with breathing in).

Call Your Doctor Now (Night or Day) If

▶ Stridor (harsh sound with breathing in) is heard now.

▶ Trouble breathing, but not severe.

▶ Lips or face have turned bluish during coughing.

▶ Breathing is much faster than normal.

▶ Can't bend the neck forward.

▶ Severe chest pain.

▶ Had croup before that needed Decadron.

▶ Weak immune system (such as sickle cell disease, HIV, cancer, organ transplant, or taking oral steroids).

▶ High-risk child (such as with cystic fibrosis or other chronic lung disease).

▶ Fever above 104°F (40°C).

▶ **Age:** Younger than 12 weeks with fever. (**Caution:** Do *not* give your baby any fever medicine before being seen.)

▶ Your child looks or acts very sick.

▶ You think your child needs to be seen, and the problem is urgent.

Call Your Doctor Within 24 Hours If

▶ Stridor (harsh sound with breathing in) occurred but not present now.

▶ Nonstop coughing.

▶ **Age:** Younger than 1 year with a croupy cough.

▶ Earache or ear drainage.

▶ Fever lasts more than 3 days.

▶ Fever returns after being gone for more than 24 hours.

▶ You think your child needs to be seen, but the problem is not urgent.

Call Your Doctor During Weekday Office Hours If

▶ Coughing causes vomiting 3 or more times.

▶ Croup is a frequent problem (3 or more times).

▶ Barky cough lasts more than 14 days.

▶ You have other questions or concerns.

Parent Care at Home If

▶ Mild croup (barky cough) with no stridor.

<h2 style="text-align:center">Care Advice 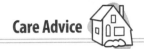</h2>

❶ What You Should Know About Croup

- Most children with croup have just a barky cough.

- Some have tight breathing (called *stridor*). Stridor is a loud, harsh sound when breathing in. It comes from the area of the voice box.

- Coughing up mucus is very important. It helps protect the lungs from pneumonia.

- We want to help a productive cough, not turn it off.

- Here is some care advice that should help.

❷ First Aid for Stridor (Harsh Sound With Breathing In) or Nonstop Coughing

- Breathe warm mist in a closed bathroom with the hot shower running. Do this for 20 minutes.

- You could also use a wet washcloth held near the face.

- **Caution:** Do not use very hot water or steam, which could cause burns.

- If warm mist fails, breathe cool air by standing near an open refrigerator. You can also go outside with your child if the weather is cold. Do this for a few minutes.

❸ Calm Your Child if Your Child Has Stridor

- Crying or fear can make stridor worse.

- Try to keep your child calm and happy.

- Hold and comfort your child.

- Use a soothing, soft voice.

❹ Humidifier

- If the air in your home is dry, use a humidifier.

- **Reason:** Dry air makes croup worse.

❺ Homemade Cough Medicine

- Coughing has a purpose. It protects the lungs. It does not need any treatment. Just keep your child well hydrated. (**Reason:** A dry throat and airway increases the coughing.) If you wish, you can also try warm fluids for bad coughing.
- **Age:** Younger than 6 months: Only give breast milk or formula.
- **Age:** 6 to 12 months. Try an ounce (30 mL) of warm water or apple juice. **Caution:** Do not use honey until 1 year of age.
- **Age:** 1 year and older. Honey is the best choice. Give ½ to 1 teaspoon (2.5–5 mL) as needed. It can thin secretions and soothe the throat. If you don't have any honey, you can use corn syrup. Can also offer warm fruit juice, herbal teas, or other clear fluid. **Amount:** A few ounces (30 mL) each time.
- **Age:** 6 years and older. Use cough drops to decrease any tickle in the throat. If you don't have any, you can use hard candy. Honey can also help. **Caution:** Avoid cough drops before 6 years. (**Reason:** Risk of choking.)

❻ Nonprescription Cough Medicine

- Nonprescription cough medicines are not advised. (**Reason:** No proven benefit for children and not approved by the US Food and Drug Administration for children younger than 6 years.)
- Honey has been shown to work better for coughs. (**Caution:** Do not use honey until 1 year of age.)
- Cough drops are a good choice after age 6.

❼ Coughing Fits or Spells: Warm Mist and Fluids

- Breathe warm mist (such as from a shower running in a closed bathroom).
- Also give warm clear fluids to drink. **Age:** Must be older than 6 months.
- **Age:** 6 to 12 months. Warm water often helps.
- **Age:** 1 year and older. Use any warm clear fluid your child likes, such as fruit juice, flavored water, or herbal teas.
- **Reason:** Warm mist and warm fluids both relax the airway and loosen up any phlegm.

❽ Fluids: Offer More

- Try to get your child to drink lots of fluids.
- **Goal:** Keep your child well hydrated.
- It also loosens up any phlegm in the lungs. Then it's easier to cough up.

❾ Fever Medicine

- For fevers above 102°F (39°C), give an acetaminophen product (such as Tylenol).

- Another choice is an ibuprofen product (such as Advil).

- **Note:** Fevers below 102°F (39°C) are important for fighting infections.

- **For all fevers:** Keep your child well hydrated. Give lots of cold fluids.

❿ Sleep Close By to Your Child

- Sleep in the same room with your child for a few nights.

- **Reason:** Stridor can start all of a sudden at night.

⓫ Avoid Tobacco Smoke

- Tobacco smoke makes croup much worse.

⓬ Return to School

- Your child can go back to school after the fever is gone.

- Your child should also feel well enough to join in normal activities.

- For practical purposes, the spread of croup and colds cannot be prevented.

⓭ What to Expect

- Most often, croup lasts 5 to 6 days and becomes worse at night.

- Croupy cough can last up to 2 weeks.

⓮ Call Your Doctor If

- Trouble breathing occurs.

- Stridor (harsh, raspy sound) occurs.

- Croupy cough lasts more than 14 days.

- You think your child needs to be seen.

- Your child becomes worse.

Remember!
Contact your doctor if your child develops any of the **Call Your Doctor** symptoms.

CHAPTER 28

Influenza, Seasonal

Definition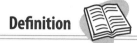

- ▶ Your child has symptoms of influenza (flu) and it's in your community.
- ▶ Main symptoms are fever AND one or more respiratory symptoms (cough, sore throat, and/or very runny nose).
- ▶ Influenza is a viral infection.
- ▶ You think your child has influenza because other family members have it OR
- ▶ You think your child has influenza because close friends have it.

Symptoms of Influenza

- ▶ Main symptoms are a fever and a runny nose, sore throat, or bad cough.
- ▶ More muscle pain, headache, fever, and chills than with usual colds.
- ▶ If there is no fever, your child probably doesn't have flu. More likely she has a cold.

Cause of Influenza

- ▶ Influenza viruses that change yearly.

Diagnosis: How to Know Your Child Has Influenza

- ▶ Influenza occurs every year in the fall and winter months. During this time, if flu symptoms occur, your child probably has the flu.
- ▶ Your child doesn't need any special tests.
- ▶ Call your doctor if your child is at high risk for complications of the flu. See next section (Children at High Risk for Complications of Influenza). She may need prescription antiviral drugs.
- ▶ For low-risk children, you don't usually need to see your child's doctor. If your child develops a possible complication of the flu, then call your doctor. See this chapter's When to Call Your Doctor section.

Children at High Risk for Complications of Influenza (American Academy of Pediatrics)

▸ Children are considered high risk if they have any of the following conditions:

- Lung disease (such as asthma).

- Heart disease (such as a congenital heart disease).

- Cancer or weak immune system.

- Neuromuscular disease (such as muscular dystrophy).

- Diabetes, sickle cell disease, kidney disease, or liver disease.

- Diseases needing long-term aspirin therapy.

- Pregnancy or severe obesity.

- Healthy children younger than 2 years are also considered high risk (Centers for Disease Control and Prevention).

▸ **Note:** All other children are referred to as *low risk.*

Prescription Antiviral Drugs for Influenza

▸ Antiviral drugs (such as Tamiflu) are sometimes used to treat influenza. They must be started within 48 hours from when the flu symptoms start. After 48 hours of fever, starting the drug is not effective.

▸ The American Academy of Pediatrics (AAP) recommends they be used for any patient with severe symptoms.

▸ The AAP recommends these drugs for most high-risk children with underlying health problems. See previous section (Children at High Risk for Complications of Influenza).

▸ The AAP doesn't recommend antiviral drugs for low-risk children with mild flu symptoms.

▸ Their benefits are limited. They usually reduce the time your child is sick by 1 to 1½ days. They also reduce symptoms, but do not make them go away.

▸ **Side effects:** Vomiting in 10% of children on Tamiflu.

▸ Most healthy children with flu do not need an antiviral drug.

When to Call Your Doctor

Call 911 Now (Your Child May Need an Ambulance) If

▶ Severe trouble breathing (struggling for each breath, can barely speak or cry).

▶ Lips or face are bluish when not coughing.

▶ You think your child has a life-threatening emergency.

Go to ER Now If

▶ Ribs are pulling in with each breath (retractions).

▶ Not alert when awake (out of it).

Call Your Doctor Now (Night or Day) If

▶ Trouble breathing, but not severe.

▶ Breathing is much faster than normal.

▶ Lips or face have turned bluish during coughing.

▶ Wheezing (tight, purring sound when breathing out).

▶ Stridor (harsh sound when breathing in).

▶ Chest pain and can't take a deep breath.

▶ Dehydration suspected (no urine in more than 8 hours, dark urine, very dry mouth, and no tears).

▶ Weak immune system (such as sickle cell disease, HIV, cancer, organ transplant, or taking oral steroids).

▶ Severe high-risk child (see this chapter's Children at High Risk for Complications of Influenza section). This includes lung disease, heart disease, and bedridden.

▶ **Age:** Younger than 12 weeks with fever. (**Caution:** Do *not* give your baby any fever medicine before being seen.)

▶ Fever above 104°F (40°C).

▶ Your child looks or acts very sick.

▶ You think your child needs to be seen, and the problem is urgent.

Call Your Doctor Within 24 Hours If

▶ Child at high risk for complications of flu. Includes children with other chronic diseases. (See this chapter's Children at High Risk for Complications of Influenza section). Also, includes healthy children younger than 2 years.

- Nonstop coughing spells.

- **Age:** Younger than 3 months with any cough.

- Earache or ear discharge.

- Sinus pain (not just congestion).

- Fever lasts more than 3 days.

- Fever returns after being gone for more than 24 hours.

- You think your child needs to be seen, but the problem is not urgent.

Call Your Doctor During Weekday Office Hours If

- **Age:** Older than 6 months and needs a flu shot.

- Coughing causes vomiting 3 or more times.

- Coughing has kept your child home from school for 3 or more days.

- Nasal discharge lasts more than 2 weeks.

- Cough lasts more than 3 weeks.

- Flu symptoms last more than 3 weeks.

- You have other questions or concerns.

Parent Care at Home If

- Influenza with no complications and your child is low risk.

Care Advice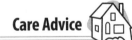

❶ What You Should Know About Influenza

- Flu symptoms include cough, sore throat, runny nose, and fever. During influenza season, if your child has these symptoms, she probably has the flu.

- Most parents know if their child has flu. They have it too or it's in the school. You don't need any special tests when you think your child has the flu.

- If your child develops a complication of the flu, then call your child's doctor. Examples are an earache or trouble breathing. These problems are included in this chapter's When to Call Your Doctor section.

- For healthy people, symptoms of influenza are like those of a bad cold.

- With flu, however, onset is more abrupt. Symptoms are more severe. Feeling very sick for the first 3 days is common.

- Treatment of influenza depends on your child's main symptoms. It is no different from treatment used for other viral colds and coughs.

- Bed rest is not needed.

- Most children with flu don't need to see their doctor.

- Here is some care advice that should help.

❷ Runny Nose With Lots of Discharge: Blow or Suction the Nose

- Nasal mucus and discharge are washing germs out the nose and sinuses.

- Blowing the nose is all that's needed. Teach your child how to blow their nose at age 2 or 3 years.

- For younger children, gently suction the nose with a suction bulb.

- Put petroleum jelly on the skin under the nose. Wash the skin first with warm water. This will help protect the nostrils from any redness.

❸ Nasal Saline Rinse to Open a Blocked Nose

- Use saline (salt water) nose spray to loosen up dried mucus. If you don't have saline, you can use a few drops of water. Use distilled water, bottled water, or boiled tap water.

  - **Step 1.** Put 3 drops in each nostril. **Age:** If younger than 1 year, use 1 drop at a time.

  - **Step 2.** Blow (or suction) each nostril out while closing off the other nostril. Then, do the other side.

  - **Step 3.** Repeat nose drops and blowing (or suctioning) until the discharge is clear.

- **How often:** Do nasal saline rinses when your child can't breathe through the nose.

- **Age:** If younger than 1 year, no more than 4 times per day. Before breast or bottle-feedings is a good time.

- Saline nose drops or spray can be bought in any drugstore. No prescription is needed.

- **Reason for nose drops:** Suction or blowing alone can't remove dried or sticky mucus. Also, babies can't breastfeed or drink from a bottle unless the nose is open.

- **Other option:** use a warm shower to loosen mucus. Breathe in the moist air and then blow each nostril.

- For young children, can also use a wet cotton swab to remove sticky mucus.

❹ Medicines for Flu

- **Cold medicines.** Don't give any drugstore cold or cough medicines to young children. They are not approved by the US Food and Drug Administration for children younger than 6 years. (**Reason:** Not safe and can cause serious side effects.) Also, they are not helpful. (**Reason:** They can't remove dried mucus from the nose.) Nasal saline rinse works best.

- **Allergy medicines.** They are not helpful unless your child also has nasal allergies. They can also help an allergic cough.

- **No antibiotics.** Antibiotics are not helpful for flu. Antibiotics may be used if your child gets an ear or sinus infection.

❺ Homemade Cough Medicine

- Coughing has a purpose. It protects the lungs. It does not need any treatment. Just keep your child well hydrated. (**Reason:** A dry throat and airway increases the coughing.) If you wish, you can also try warm fluids for bad coughing.

- **Age:** Younger than 6 months: Only give breast milk or formula.

- **Age:** 6 to 12 months. Try an ounce (30 mL) of warm water or apple juice. **Caution:** Do not use honey until 1 year of age.

- **Age:** 1 year and older. Honey is the best choice. Give ½ to 1 teaspoon (2.5–5 mL) as needed. It can thin secretions and soothe the throat. If you don't have any honey, you can use corn syrup. Can also offer warm fruit juice, herbal teas, or other clear fluid. **Amount:** A few ounces (30 mL) each time.

- **Age:** 6 years and older. Use cough drops to decrease any tickle in the throat. If you don't have any, you can use hard candy. Honey can also help. **Caution:** Avoid cough drops before 6 years. (**Reason:** Risk of choking.)

❻ Sore Throat Pain Relief

- **Age:** Older than 1 year. Can sip warm fluids, such as chicken broth or apple juice. Some children prefer cold foods such as Popsicles or ice cream.

- **Age:** Older than 6 years. Can also suck on hard candy or lollipops. Butterscotch seems to help.

- **Age:** Older than 8 years. Can also gargle. Use warm water with a little table salt added. A liquid antacid can be added instead of salt. Use Mylanta or the store brand. No prescription is needed.

- Medicated throat sprays or lozenges are generally not helpful.

❼ Fluids: Offer More

- Try to get your child to drink lots of fluids.
- **Goal:** Keep your child well hydrated.
- It will also thin out mucus discharge from the nose.
- It also loosens up any phlegm in the lungs. Then it's easier to cough up.

❽ Fever Medicine

- For fevers above 102°F (39°C), give an acetaminophen product (such as Tylenol).
- Another choice is an ibuprofen product (such as Advil).
- Avoid aspirin because of the strong link with Reye syndrome.
- **Note:** Fevers below 102°F (39°C) are important for fighting infections.
- **For all fevers:** Keep your child well hydrated. Give lots of cold fluids.

❾ Pain Medicine

- For muscle aches or headaches, give an acetaminophen product (such as Tylenol).
- Another choice is an ibuprofen product (such as Advil).
- Use as needed.

❿ Prescription Antiviral Drugs for Influenza

- Antiviral drugs (such as Tamiflu) are sometimes used to treat influenza. They must be started within 48 hours from when flu symptoms start. After 48 hours of fever, starting the drug is not effective.
- The AAP recommends they be used for any patient with severe symptoms. They also recommend these drugs for most high-risk children. See this chapter's Children at High Risk for Complications of Influenza section.
- If your child has a chronic disease and gets the flu, call your doctor. The doctor will decide if your child needs a prescription.
- The AAP doesn't recommend antiviral drugs for low-risk children with normal flu symptoms.
- Benefits are limited. They reduce the time your child is sick by 1 to 1½ days. They also reduce symptoms but do not make them go away.
- **Side effects:** Vomiting in 10% of children on Tamiflu.
- Most healthy children with flu do not need an antiviral drug.

- Also, it is not used to prevent flu. (**Reason:** You would need to take the medicine every day for months).

⑪ Return to School

- Spread is rapid, and the virus is easily passed to others.
- The time it takes to get the flu after contact is about 2 days.
- Your child can return to school after the fever is gone for 24 hours.
- Your child should feel well enough to join in normal activities.

⑫ What to Expect

- Influenza causes a cough that lasts 2 to 3 weeks.
- Sometimes your child will cough up lots of phlegm (mucus). The mucus can be gray, yellow, or green. This is normal.
- Coughing up mucus is very important. It helps protect the lungs from pneumonia.
- We want to help a productive cough, not turn it off.
- Fever lasts 2 to 3 days.
- Runny nose lasts 7 to 14 days.

⑬ Prevention: How to Protect Yourself From Getting Sick

- Wash hands often with soap and water.
- Alcohol-based hand cleaners also work well.
- Avoid touching the eyes, nose, or mouth. Germs on the hands can spread this way.
- Try to avoid close contact with sick people.
- Avoid ERs and urgent care centers if you don't need to go. These are places where you are more likely to be exposed to the flu.

⑭ Prevention/How to Protect Others: Stay Home When Sick

- Cover the nose and mouth with a tissue when coughing or sneezing.
- Wash hands often with soap and water, especially after coughing or sneezing.
- Limit contact with others to keep from infecting them.
- Stay home from school for at least 24 hours after the fever is gone (Centers for Disease Control and Prevention).

ⓕ Flu Shot and Prevention

- Getting a flu shot is the best way to protect your family from flu.

- Influenza vaccines are strongly advised for all children older than 6 months (AAP).

- Adults should also get the shot.

- The shot most often prevents the disease.

- Even if your child gets the flu, the shot helps reduce symptoms.

- A new flu shot is needed every year. (**Reason:** Flu viruses keep changing.)

- It takes 2 weeks to be fully protected from flu after the flu shot. The protection lasts for the full flu season. An antiviral medicine protects from flu only while taking it.

ⓖ Call Your Doctor If

- Trouble breathing occurs.

- Retractions (pulling in between the ribs) occur.

- Dehydration occurs.

- Earache or sinus pain occurs.

- Fever lasts more than 3 days or goes above 104°F (40°C).

- Nasal discharge lasts more than 14 days.

- Cough lasts more than 3 weeks.

- You think your child needs to be seen.

- Your child becomes worse.

Remember!
Contact your doctor if your child develops any of the **Call Your Doctor** symptoms.

CHAPTER 29

COVID-19, Diagnosed or Suspected

Definition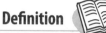

- ▶ Your child has a COVID-19 viral infection.
- ▶ The diagnosis was confirmed by a positive laboratory test result.
- ▶ If COVID-19 is suspected, always get a laboratory test to know for sure.

Symptoms of COVID-19

- ▶ The most common symptoms are cough and fever. Some people progress to shortness of breath and trouble breathing.
- ▶ Other common symptoms are runny nose, chills, shivering (shaking), sore throat, muscle pains or body aches, headache, fatigue (tiredness), and loss of smell or taste.
- ▶ The Centers for Disease Control and Prevention (CDC) also includes the following less common symptoms: nausea, vomiting, and diarrhea.

COVID-19 Facts

- ▶ **Incubation period.** Average: 5 days (range: 2–10 days) after coming in contact with the secretions of a person who has COVID-19.
- ▶ **Spread.** The virus spreads when respiratory droplets are produced as a person coughs, sneezes, shouts, or sings. The infected droplets can then be inhaled by a nearby person. These are how most respiratory viruses spread.
- ▶ **No symptoms, but infected.** More than 30% of infected people have no symptoms.
- ▶ **Mild infections.** Eighty percent of those with symptoms have a mild illness, much like normal flu or a bad cold. The symptoms usually last 1 to 2 weeks.
- ▶ **Severe infections.** Twenty percent of those with symptoms develop some trouble breathing. Some of these people need to be admitted to the hospital.
- ▶ **Vaccine.** Safe and highly effective vaccines are available. The vaccine prevents almost all hospital admissions and deaths. Any breakthrough infections are usually mild.
- ▶ **Treatment.** Special treatments are also available for severe COVID-19.

When to Call Your Doctor

Call 911 Now (Your Child May Need an Ambulance) If

▸ Severe trouble breathing (struggling for each breath, can barely speak).

▸ Lips or face are bluish now.

▸ You think your child has a life-threatening emergency.

Call Your Doctor Now (Night or Day) If

▸ Trouble breathing, but not severe (includes tight breathing and hard breathing).

▸ Ribs are pulling in with each breath (called *retractions*).

▸ Breathing is much faster than normal.

▸ Lips or face have turned bluish during coughing.

▸ Wheezing (tight, purring sound with breathing out).

▸ Stridor (harsh sound with breathing in).

▸ Chest pain or pressure and can't take a deep breath.

▸ Sore throat with serious symptoms (such as can't swallow fluids or has new-onset drooling).

▸ Muscle pains with serious symptoms (such as can't walk or can barely walk).

▸ Headache with serious symptoms (such as worst headache ever, confusion, weakness, or stiff neck).

▸ Dehydration suspected. No urine in over 8 hours, dark urine, very dry mouth, and no tears.

▸ Weak immune system, such as HIV, cancer, organ transplant, or taking oral steroids.

▸ High-risk child. This includes with lung disease, heart disease, diabetes, or other serious chronic disease.

▸ Age: Younger than 12 weeks with fever.

▸ Fever above 104°F (40°C).

▸ Your child looks or acts very sick.

▸ You think your child needs to be seen, and the problem is urgent.

Call Your Doctor Within 24 Hours If

► Nonstop coughing spells.

► Age: Younger than 3 months with any cough.

► Earache or ear discharge.

► Sinus pain (not just congestion).

► Fever lasts more than 3 days.

► Fever returns after gone for more than 24 hours.

► You think your child needs to be seen, but the problem is not urgent.

Parent Care at Home If

► Diagnosed or suspected COVID-19 with mild symptoms.

Care Advice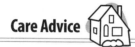

❶ Treatment of Symptoms

■ The treatment is the same whether your child has COVID-19, influenza, or some other respiratory viral infection.

■ The only difference for COVID-19 is the need to stay on home isolation until your child recovers. (**Reason:** You want to protect other people from getting it.) The elderly and people with serious health problems can die from COVID-19.

■ Treat the symptoms that are bothering your child the most. See Chapter 28, Influenza, Seasonal, for details of home treatment.

■ There is no antiviral medicine for treating mild COVID-19 in healthy, low-risk children.

■ Antibiotics are not helpful for viral infections.

■ You don't need to call or see your doctor unless your child develops trouble breathing or becomes worse in any other way.

❷ Call Your Doctor If

■ Shortness of breath occurs.

■ Trouble breathing occurs.

■ Your child becomes worse.

COVID-19 Home Isolation Questions

❶ Home Isolation Is Needed for Those Who Are Sick

- Isolation means separating sick people with a contagious disease from people who are not sick (CDC). That means stay at home.

- Your child does not need to be confined to a single room. Preventing spread of respiratory infections within a home is nearly impossible. But try to avoid very close contact with other family members, such as hugging, kissing, sitting next to, or sleeping in the same bed as each other. Other family members should also stay at home on quarantine. **Reason:** Living with a suspected COVID-19 person implies that close contact has occurred.

- Do not allow your child any visitors (such as friends).

- Do not send your child to school.

- Do not go to stores, restaurants, places of worship, or other public places.

❷ Stopping Home Isolation: Must Meet All 3 Requirements (CDC)

- Fever gone for at least 24 hours after stopping fever-reducing medicines AND

- Cough and other symptoms must be improved AND

- Symptoms started more than 5 days ago.

- Summary: You must isolate at home for at least 5 days. Then wear a mask around others for another 5 days. If your child is too young to wear a mask, they need to stay home for 10 days.

- If you're unsure about whether it is safe for you to leave isolation, check the CDC website or call your doctor.

COVID-19 Prevention

❶ COVID-19 Vaccine: Get Your COVID-19 Shot

- Vaccines have saved more lives than any other public health action. They are the most powerful weapon we have against deadly infectious diseases. Follow the science.

- Safe and highly effective vaccines are available. Get the vaccine per the CDC and AAP recommendations. It could save your life and protect your family.

❷ COVID-19: How to Protect Yourself and Family From Catching It—The Basics

- Wash hands often with soap and water (very important). Always do this before you eat.

- Use an alcohol-based hand sanitizer if water is not available. Remember, soap and water work better.

- Don't touch your eyes, nose, or mouth unless your hands are clean. Germs on the hands can get into your body this way.

❸ Social (Safe) Distancing and COVID-19 Prevention

- Avoid any contact with people known to have COVID-19.

- **Social distancing.** Try to stay at least 6 feet (2 meters) away from anyone who is sick, especially if they are coughing. Avoid crowds within your community, because you can't tell who might be sick.

❹ Face Masks and COVID-19 Prevention

- **Overview.** Face masks are helpful for reducing the spread of COVID-19. **Reason:** People with COVID-19 can have no symptoms but still spread the virus. Masks also reduce the spread of flu.

- Follow the CDC recommendations on when to wear masks.

❺ Breastfeeding if Mother Has COVID-19

- Breastfeeding experts recommend that you continue to breastfeed even if you are sick with COVID-19.

- Wash your hands before feeding your baby.

- The CDC recommends wearing a face mask if you are sick. Be careful to avoid coughing on your baby.

- Breast milk gives beneficial antibodies that your body is making against this illness to your baby. This should provide some protection against this illness for your baby, as it does for influenza and most other viral illnesses.

- Research has proven that the virus is not passed through breast milk.

- Breastfeeding mothers should also get the COVID-19 vaccine (CDC).

Remember!
Contact your doctor if your child develops any of the **Call Your Doctor** symptoms.

CHAPTER 30
Coughs and Colds: Medicines or Home Remedies?

Medicines (Over-the-counter)

▶ Over-the-counter cough and cold medicines can cause side effects. These side effects can be serious in young children. Risks of using these medicines outweigh any benefits. In 2008, the US Food and Drug Administration looked at this issue in children. They recommended these medicines never be used in young children. After age 6, the medicines are safe to use if you follow the package instructions. But, it's easy to treat coughs and colds without these medicines.

Home Remedies

▶ A good home remedy is safe, cheap, and as helpful as over-the-counter medicines. Home remedies are also found in nearly every home. Here are some simple but helpful home treatments.

❶ Runny Nose: Suction or Blow the Nose

■ When your child's nose runs like a faucet, it's getting rid of the virus. Teach your child how to blow their nose at age 2 or 3 years. Allergy medicines (such as Benadryl) do not help the average cold. They are useful only if your child has nasal allergies (hay fever).

❷ Blocked Nose: Use a Nasal Saline Rinse

■ Use saline (salt water) nose drops or spray to loosen up dried mucus. If you don't have saline, you can use a few drops of water. Use distilled water, bottled water, or boiled tap water.

– **Step 1.** Put 3 drops in each nostril. If younger than 1 year, use 1 drop.

– **Step 2.** Blow (or suction) each nostril separately, while closing off the other nostril. Then do the other side.

– **Step 3.** Repeat nose drops and blowing (or suctioning) until the discharge is clear.

■ **How often:** Do nasal saline rinses when your child can't breathe through the nose.

■ **Limit:** If younger than 1 year, no more than 4 times per day or before every feeding.

- Saline nose drops or spray can be bought in any drugstore. No prescription is needed.

- **Reason for nose drops:** Suction or blowing alone can't remove dried or sticky mucus. Also, babies can't breastfeed or drink from a bottle unless the nose is open.

- **Other option:** Use a warm shower to loosen mucus. Breathe in the moist air and then blow (or suction) each nostril.

- For young children, can also use a wet cotton swab to remove sticky mucus.

- **Medicines:** No drugs can remove dried mucus from the nose.

❸ Coughing: Use Homemade Cough Medicines

- Coughing has a purpose. It protects the lungs. It does not need any treatment. Just keep your child well hydrated. (**Reason:** A dry throat and airway increases the coughing.) If you wish, you can also try warm fluids for bad coughing.

- **Age:** Younger than 6 months: Only give breast milk or formula.

- **Age:** 6 to 12 months. Try an ounce (30 mL) of warm water or apple juice. **Caution:** Do not use honey until 1 year of age.

- **Age:** 1 year and older. Honey is the best choice. Give ½ to 1 teaspoon (2.5–5 mL) as needed. It can thin secretions and soothe the throat. If you don't have any honey, you can use corn syrup. Can also offer warm fruit juice, herbal teas, or other clear fluid. **Amount:** A few ounces (30 mL) each time.

- **Age:** 6 years and older. Use cough drops to decrease any tickle in the throat. If you don't have any, you can use hard candy. Honey can also help. **Caution:** Avoid cough drops before 6 years. (**Reason:** Risk of choking.)

- **Coughing fits:** Warm mist from a hot shower can help.

❹ Fluids: Help Your Child Drink Lots of Fluids

- Staying well hydrated thins the body's secretions. That makes it easier to cough and blow the nose.

❺ Humidity

- If the air in your home is dry, use a humidifier. Moist air keeps the nose and airway from drying out. Run a warm shower for a while to help put moisture in the air.

Treatment Is Not Always Needed

- If symptoms aren't bothering your child, he doesn't need medicine or any treatment. Many children with a cough or cold are happy, play fine, and sleep well.

- Treat symptoms only if they cause discomfort or wake your child up. Treat a cough if it's hacking and really bothers your child.

- Fevers are helpful. Treat them only if they slow your child down or cause some discomfort. That does not occur until 102°F (39°C) or higher. Acetaminophen (Tylenol) or ibuprofen (Motrin or Advil) can be given. Use to treat higher fever or pain. See drug dosage charts in the Appendix.

Summary

If coughs or colds need treatment, home remedies may work better than medicines.

CHAPTER 31

Antibiotics: When Do They Help?

Definition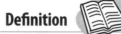

▶ Antibiotics are strong medicines that can kill bacteria. They have saved many lives and prevented bad complications. These drugs do not kill viruses. They work only on bacteria. Every day, doctors must decide if a child's infection is viral or bacterial. Here's how they do it.

Bacterial Infections

▶ Much less common than viral infections. Antibiotics can help. Bacteria cause

- Some ear infections.

- Most sinus infections (not sinus congestion).

- Twenty percent of sore throats, which are strep throat infections.

- Ten percent of pneumonias (a lung infection).

Viral Infections

▶ Most infections in children are caused by a virus. Antibiotics do not help. Viruses cause

- 100% of colds. (**Note:** Unless they turn into an ear or sinus infection. This happens with 5%–10% of colds.)

- 95% of new coughs. (**Note:** Asthma can also start with a cough.)

- 95% of fevers.

- 80% of sore throats.

- 90% of pneumonia. (**Note:** Most cases in children are caused by a virus.)

- 99% of diarrhea and vomiting.

- **Note:** A few antiviral drugs can treat viral infections. An example is Tamiflu, used for severe influenza.

Cold Symptoms That Are Normal

▸ Parents are sometimes worried about common cold symptoms. The symptoms below are not signs of bacterial infections. Nor are they a reason to start antibiotics.

- **Green or yellow nose discharge.** This is a normal part of getting over a cold. It is not a clue of a sinus infection.

- **Green or yellow coughed-up phlegm.** This is a normal part of getting over viral bronchitis. It is not a sign of pneumonia.

- **High fevers.** High fevers (above 104°F or 40°C) can be caused by a virus or bacteria.

Side Effects of Antibiotics

▸ All antibiotics have side effects. Some children taking these drugs experience side effects. Examples are diarrhea, nausea, vomiting, or a rash. Loose stools occur because the drug kills off good bacteria in the gut. If your child gets a rash, it can be from the drug. Your doctor has to decide if the rash is an allergy. The biggest side effect of overuse is called *antibiotic resistance*. This is when the germs are no longer killed by the drug. That's why we use antibiotics only if a child really needs them.

Giving Antibiotics for Viral Infections: What Happens?

▸ If your child has a virus, an antibiotic won't get rid of the fever. It will not help the other symptoms. The drug will not get your child back to school or you back to work any faster. If your child has side effects from the drug, she will feel worse.

What You Can Do

▸ Save antibiotics for bacterial infections when your child really needs them.

▸ Don't pressure your child's doctor for an antibiotic.

▸ Treat your child's cold and cough symptoms with home treatment that works.

▸ Keep in mind that fever is fighting the infection. It also boosts the immune system to prevent future infections.

PART 8

Abdominal Symptoms

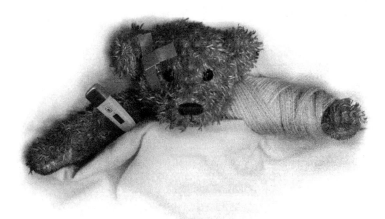

CHAPTER 32

Abdominal Pain

Definition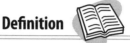

- Pain or discomfort in the stomach (belly) area.
- Pain found between bottom of the rib cage and groin crease.
- The older child reports stomach pain.
- The younger child points to or holds the stomach.

See Other Chapter If

- Stomach pain and younger than 12 months or crying and you are not sure what it causing it. See Chapter 7, Crying Child.
- Constipation is the main symptom. See Chapter 33, Constipation.
- Diarrhea is the main symptom. See Chapter 34, Diarrhea.
- Vomiting (or child feels like he needs to vomit) is the main symptom. See Chapter 36, Vomiting Without Diarrhea.
- Passing urine is painful and stomach pain is mild. See Chapter 37, Urination Pain.

Causes of Acute Stomach Pain

- **Eating too much.** Eating too much can cause an upset stomach and mild stomach pain.
- **Hunger pains.** Younger children may report stomach pain when they are hungry.
- **Gastrointestinal (GI) virus (such as *Rotavirus*).** A GI virus can cause stomach cramps as well as vomiting or diarrhea.
- **Food poisoning.** This causes sudden vomiting or diarrhea within hours after eating the bad food. It is caused by toxins from germs growing in foods left out too long. Most often, symptoms go away in less than 24 hours. It can often be treated at home without the need for medical care.

▸ **Constipation.** The need to pass a stool may cause cramps in the lower abdomen.

▸ **Strep throat.** A strep throat infection causes 10% of new-onset stomach pain with fever.

▸ **Bladder infection.** Bladder infections usually present with painful urination, urgency, and bad-smelling urine. Sometimes the only symptom is pain in the lower abdomen.

▸ **Appendicitis (serious).** Suspect appendicitis if pain is low on the right side and your child walks bent over. Other signs are a child who won't hop and wants to lie still.

▸ **Intussusception (serious).** Sudden attacks of severe pain that switch back and forth with periods of calm. Caused by one segment of bowel telescoping into a lower piece of bowel. Peak age is 6 months to 2 years.

Causes of Recurrent Stomach Pains

▸ **Stress or worries.** The most common cause of frequent stomach pains is stress. More than 10% of children have a "worried stomach." These children tend to be sensitive and too serious. They are often model children. This can make them more at risk to the normal stresses of life. Examples of these events are changing schools, moving, or family disagreements. Pain is in the pit of the stomach or near the belly button. The pain is real.

▸ **Abdominal migraine.** Attacks of stomach pain and vomiting with sudden onset and offset. Often occur in children who later develop migraines. Strongly genetic.

▸ **Functional abdominal pains.** Functional means stomach pains are due to a sensitive GI tract. The GI tract is free of any disease.

▸ **School avoidance.** Stomach pains that mainly occur in the morning on school days. They keep a child from going to school.

Pain Scale

▸ **Mild:** Your child feels pain and tells you about it. The pain does not keep your child from doing any normal activities. School, play, and sleep are not changed.

▸ **Moderate:** The pain keeps your child from doing some normal activities. It may wake your child up from sleep.

▸ **Severe:** The pain is very bad. It keeps your child from doing all normal activities.

When to Call Your Doctor

Call 911 Now (Your Child May Need an Ambulance) If

▶ Not moving or too weak to stand.

▶ You think your child has a life-threatening emergency.

Go to ER Now If

▶ Appendicitis suspected (pain low on right side, won't jump, wants to lie still).

▶ Severe, constant pain (child not able to move or do anything).

▶ Can't walk or walks bent over holding the stomach.

▶ Blood in the stool or vomiting blood.

▶ Vomiting bile (green color). (**Exception:** Stomach juice that is yellow.)

▶ Swallowed object (such as a coin) suspected.

Call Your Doctor Now (Night or Day) If

▶ Pain low on the right side.

▶ Pain or swelling in the scrotum (male).

▶ Could be pregnant (female).

▶ Constant pain (or crying) for more than 2 hours.

▶ Recent injury to the stomach.

▶ High-risk child (such as with diabetes, sickle cell disease, or recent abdominal surgery).

▶ **Age:** Younger than 2 years.

▶ Fever above 104°F (40°C).

▶ Your child looks or acts very sick.

▶ You think your child needs to be seen, and the problem is urgent.

Call Your Doctor Within 24 Hours If

▶ Moderate pain keeps your child from doing some normal activities.

▶ Mild pain comes and goes (cramps) but lasts more than 24 hours.

▶ Fever is present.

▸ Bladder infection (UTI [urinary tract infection]) suspected (passing urine hurts, new-onset wetting).

▸ You think your child needs to be seen, but the problem is not urgent.

Call Your Doctor During Weekday Office Hours If

▸ Stomach pains are a frequent problem.

▸ You have other questions or concerns.

Parent Care at Home If

▸ Mild stomach pain.

Care Advice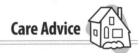

❶ What You Should Know About Stomach Pain

■ Mild stomach pain can be caused by something simple. It could be from gas pains or eating too much.

■ Sometimes, stomach pain signals the start of a viral infection. This will lead to vomiting or loose stools.

■ Watching your child for 2 hours will help tell you the cause.

■ Here is some care advice that should help.

❷ Lie Down

■ Have your child lie down and rest until feeling better.

❸ Clear Fluids

■ Offer only clear fluids (such as water, flat soft drinks, or half-strength sports drinks such as Gatorade).

■ For mild pain, offer a regular diet.

❹ Prepare for Vomiting

■ Keep a vomiting pan handy.

■ Younger children often talk about stomach pain when they have nausea. Nausea is the sick stomach feeling that comes before throwing up.

❺ Pass a Stool

- Have your child sit on the toilet and try to pass a stool.
- This may help if pain is from constipation or diarrhea.
- **Note:** For constipation, moving a warm, wet cotton ball over the anus may help.

❻ Do Not Give Medicines

- Any drug (like ibuprofen) could upset the stomach and make pain worse.
- Do not give any pain medicines or laxatives for stomach cramps.
- For fever above 102°F (39°C), acetaminophen (such as Tylenol) can be given.

❼ What to Expect

- With harmless causes, pain is most often better or gone in 2 hours.
- With stomach flu, belly cramps may happen before each bout of vomiting or diarrhea. These cramps may come and go for a few days.
- With serious causes (such as appendicitis), pain worsens and becomes constant.

❽ Call Your Doctor If

- Pain becomes severe.
- Constant pain lasts more than 2 hours.
- Mild pain comes and goes and lasts more than 24 hours.
- You think your child needs to be seen.
- Your child becomes worse.

❾ Extra Help: Worried Stomach

- Help your child talk about events that trigger stomach pain. Talk with your child about how to cope with these the next time around.
- Help your child worry less about things he can't control.
- To treat pain, help your child get very relaxed. Lying down in a quiet place and taking slow, deep breaths may help. Make the belly go up and down with each breath. Then try to relax all the muscles in the body. Think about something pleasant. Listening to audio that teaches how to relax might also help.

- Make sure your child gets enough sleep.

- Make sure your child doesn't miss any school because of stomach pains. Stressed children tend to want to stay home when the going gets rough.

- **Caution:** Your child should see a doctor for an examination. Do this before concluding frequent stomach pains are from worrying too much.

Remember!
Contact your doctor if your child develops any of the **Call Your Doctor** symptoms.

CHAPTER 33

Constipation

Definition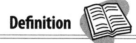

- Can't pass a stool or pain when passing a stool (bowel movement).

- Crying when passing a stool, or passing a stool after straining or pushing longer than 10 minutes.

- Three or more days without passing a stool. (**Exception:** Breastfed and older than 1 month.)

- **Caution:** Any belly pain from constipation comes and goes. Most often, it is mild. See Chapter 32, Abdominal Pain, if there is constant belly pain.

See Other Chapter If

- Constant belly pain. See Chapter 31, Abdominal Pain.

- Doesn't meet the definition of constipation and older than 1 year.

Causes of Constipation

- **High cow's milk diet.** Milk and cheese are the only foods that in high amounts can cause constipation. They cause hard pale stools. This is why you want your child to eat a well-balanced diet.

- **Low-fiber diet.** Fiber is found in vegetables, fruits, and whole grains. Fiber keeps stools soft, bulky, and easy to pass. A low-fiber diet causes hard, small stools.

- **Low fluid intake.** This can also cause stools to be dry and harder to pass. It's rarely the only cause of constipation.

- **Lack of exercise.** Exercise also keeps the bowel from slowing down. Not a cause in children unless they are on bed rest.

- **Holding back stools because of pain.** If passing a stool causes pain, many children will hold back the next one. This can happen with a strep infection around the anus. It can also occur with a bad diaper rash or anal fissure (tear).

- **Holding back stools because of power struggles.** This is the most common cause of recurrent constipation in children. Most often it's a battle around toilet training. If children are already trained, it may begin with the start of school. (**Reason:** Some children refuse to use public toilets. Some children postpone stools because they are too busy to sit down.)

- **Slow passage** of food through the intestines. Most often, this type runs in families. Called *slow transit time*.

Stools: How Often Is Normal?

- **Normal range:** 3 per day to 1 every 2 days. Once children are on normal table foods, their stool pattern is like adults.

- Kids who go every 4 or 5 days almost always have pain with passage. They also have a lot of straining.

- Kids who go every 3 days often drift into longer times. Then, they also develop symptoms.

- Passing a stool should be free of pain.

- Any child with pain during stool passage or lots of straining needs treatment. At the very least, the child should be treated with changes in diet.

Imitators of Constipation: Normal Patterns and Stools

- **Breastfed and older than 1 month.** Stools every 4 to 7 days that are soft, large, and pain-free can be normal. (**Caution:** Before 1 month of age, not stooling enough can mean not getting enough breast milk.)

- **Straining in babies.** Grunting or straining while pushing out a stool is normal in young babies. They are learning to relax their anus after 9 months of keeping it closed. It's also hard for them to pass stool lying on their back with no help from gravity. Babies also become red in the face and draw up their legs during straining. This is normal.

- **Brief straining** fewer than 10 minutes can occur at times at any age.

- **Large stools.** Size relates to the amount of food eaten. Large eaters have larger stools.

- **Hard or dry stools.** Also can be normal if passed easily without too much straining. Often, this relates to poor fiber intake. Some children even have small, dry rabbit pellet–like stools.

When to Call Your Doctor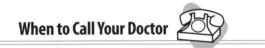

Go to ER Now If

- Vomiting bile (green color). (**Exception:** Stomach juice that is yellow.)

Call Your Doctor Now (Night or Day) If

▶ Stomach pain persists for more than 1 hour (includes crying) after using this chapter's Care Advice.

▶ Rectal pain lasts more than 1 hour (includes straining) after using this chapter's Care Advice.

▶ Vomits 2 or more times and stomach looks more swollen than normal.

▶ **Age:** Younger than 1 month and breastfed.

▶ **Age:** Younger than 12 months with recent onset of weak suck or weak muscles.

▶ Your child looks or acts very sick.

▶ You think your child needs to be seen, and the problem is urgent.

Call Your Doctor Within 24 Hours If

▶ **Age:** Younger than 2 months. (**Exception:** Normal straining and grunting.)

▶ Bleeding from anus.

▶ Needs to pass a stool but afraid to or refuses to let it out.

▶ Child may be blocked up.

▶ Suppository or enema was given but did not work.

▶ You think your child needs to be seen, but the problem is not urgent.

Call Your Doctor During Weekday Office Hours If

▶ Leaking stool.

▶ Suppository or enema was needed to get the stool out.

▶ Infrequent stools do not get better after changes to diet. (**Exception:** Normal if breastfed infant older than 1 month and stools are not painful.)

▶ Stool softeners are being used and have not been discussed with your doctor.

▶ Toilet training is in progress.

▶ Painful stools occur 3 or more times after changes to diet.

▶ Constipation is a frequent problem.

▶ You have other questions or concerns.

Parent Care at Home If

▶ Mild constipation.

Care Advice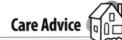

❶ What You Should Know About Constipation

- Constipation is common in children.

- Most often, it's from a change in diet. It can also be caused by waiting too long to pass a stool.

- Passing a stool should be pleasant and free of pain.

- Any child with pain during stool passage or lots of straining needs treatment. At the very least, she need changes in diet.

- Here is some care advice that should help.

❷ Normal Stools

- Normal range: 3 per day to 1 every 2 days. Once children are on a regular diet, their stool pattern is like adults.

- Kids who go every 3 days often drift into longer times. Then symptoms start.

- Kids who go every 4 and 5 days almost always have pain with passage. They also have lots of straining.

❸ Diet for Babies Younger Than 1 Year

- **Age:** Older than 1 month and only on breast milk or formula. Add fruit juice. **Amount:** Give 1 ounce (30 mL) per month of age per day. Limit amount to 4 ounces (120 mL). Pear and apple juice are good options. After 3 months, can use prune (plum) juice. (**Reason:** Fruit juice is approved for babies to treat a symptom.)

- **Age:** Older than 4 months. Also add baby foods with high fiber. Do this twice a day. Examples are peas, beans, apricots, prunes, peaches, pears, or plums.

- **Age:** Older than 8 months on finger foods. Add cereals and small pieces of fresh fruit.

❹ Diet for Children Older Than 1 Year

- Increase fruit juice (apple, pear, cherry, grape, prune). (**Note:** Citrus fruit juices are not helpful.)

- Add fruits and vegetables high in fiber content. Examples are peas, beans, broccoli, bananas, apricots, peaches, pears, figs, prunes, or dates. Offer these foods 3 or more times per day.

- Increase whole grain foods. Examples are bran flakes or muffins, graham crackers, and oatmeal. Brown rice and whole wheat bread are also helpful. Popcorn can be used if older than 4 years.

- Limit milk products (milk, ice cream, cheese, yogurt) to 3 servings per day.

- **Fluids:** Give enough fluids to stay well hydrated. (**Reason:** Keeps the stool soft.)

❺ Stop Toilet Training

- Put your child back in diapers or Pull-Ups for a short time.

- Tell her that the poops won't hurt when they come out.

- Praise her for passing poops into a diaper.

- Holding back stools is harmful. Use rewards to help your child give up this bad habit.

- Avoid any pressure or punishment. Also, never force your child to sit on the potty against her will. (**Reason:** It will cause a power struggle.)

- Treats and hugs always work better than punishment.

❻ Encourage Sitting on the Toilet (if Toilet Trained)

- Set up a normal stool routine if your child agrees to sitting.

- Have your child sit on the toilet for 5 minutes after meals.

- This is especially important after breakfast.

- If you see your child holding back a stool, if they cooperate, take them to the toilet to sit.

- During sitting, stay with your child and be a coach. Focus on helping the stool come out.

- Do not distract your child. Do not allow your child to play with video devices, games, or books while on the toilet.

- Once she passes a normal-sized stool, she doesn't need to sit anymore that day.

❼ Warm Water to Relax the Anus

- Warmth helps many children relax the anus and release a stool.

- For straining too long, have your child sit in warm water.

- You can also put a warm, wet cotton ball on the anus. Vibrate it side to side for about 10 seconds to help relax the anus.

❽ Flexed Position to Help Stool Release for Babies

- Help your baby by holding the knees against the chest. This is like squatting for your baby. This is the natural position for pushing out a stool. It's hard to pass a stool lying down.

- Gently pumping the left side of the belly also helps.

❾ Squatting Position to Help Stool Release for Older Children

- The squatting position gives faster stool release and less straining.
- Squatting means that the knees are above the hips.
- For most children who sit on the toilet, a footstool is needed.
- It is an important part of treating constipation.

❿ Stool Softeners (Age: Older Than 1 Year)

- If a change in diet doesn't help, you can add a stool softener. Must be older than 1 year.
- Use a stool softener (such as Miralax). It is available without a prescription. Give 1 to 3 teaspoons (5–15 mL) powder each day with dinner. Mix each teaspoon (5 mL) of powder with 2 ounces (60 mL) of water.
- Fiber products (such as Benefiber) are also helpful. Give 1 teaspoon (5 mL) twice a day. Mix it in 2 ounces (60 mL) of water or fruit juice.
- Stool softeners and fiber should produce regular soft stools in 1 to 3 days.
- Discuss dosage and how long to use with your doctor.

⓫ What to Expect

- Most often, changes in diet help constipation.
- After your child is better, be sure to keep her on high-fiber foods.
- Also, have your child sit on the toilet at the same time each day.
- These tips will help prevent symptoms from coming back.

⓬ Call Your Doctor If

- Constipation lasts more than 1 week after making changes to diet.
- You think your child needs to be seen.
- Your child becomes worse.

Remember!
Contact your doctor if your child develops any of the **Call Your Doctor** symptoms.

CHAPTER 34

Diarrhea

Definition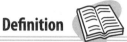

- ► Sudden increase in number and looseness of stools.

- ► Diarrhea means 3 or more watery or very loose stools. (**Reason:** 1 or 2 loose stools can be normal with changes in diet.)

See Other Chapter If

- ► Vomiting along with loose stools. See Chapter 35, Vomiting With Diarrhea.

Causes of Acute Diarrhea

- ► **Virus** (such as *Rotavirus*). An infection of the intestines from a virus is the most common cause.

- ► **Bacteria** (such as *Salmonella*). Less common cause. Diarrhea often contains streaks of blood.

- ► **Food poisoning.** This causes rapid vomiting and diarrhea within hours after eating the bad food. It is caused by toxins from germs growing in foods left out too long. Most often, symptoms go away in less than 24 hours. It can often be treated at home without the need for medical care.

- ► **Giardia** (a parasite). More likely in child care center outbreaks.

- ► **Traveler's diarrhea.** Caused by germs in food or drink. Suspect this if it follows recent foreign travel.

- ► **Antibiotic diarrhea.** Many antibiotics cause mild diarrhea. This is not an allergic reaction. Keep giving the antibiotic. Call your doctor if any serious symptoms occur.

- ► **Serious causes.** Most bacterial diarrhea goes away on its own. A few can cause a severe, large bowel infection (such as *Shigella* colitis). *Clostridium difficile* is a serious cause that can occur after being on strong antibiotics.

- ► **Serious complication: dehydration.** This is the health problem for which the body has lost too much fluid. (See this chapter's Dehydration: How to Know section.)

Causes of Recurrent Diarrhea

▸ **Cow's milk allergy.** Can cause loose, slimy stools in babies. Can be blood streaked. Starts within the first 2 months of life. Need to avoid cow's milk formulas.

▸ **Toddler's diarrhea.** Toddlers who pass 3 to 6 runny stools per day. Stools may run out of the diaper. Symptoms begin at age 1 year. Symptoms resolve at age 3 or 4, after being toilet trained. Harmless and no effect on growth. Fruit juice makes it worse. The cause is rapid transit time from stomach to anus. May develop irritable bowel syndrome in adult years.

▸ **Lactose intolerance.** Lactose is the sugar in milk. Many people cannot absorb lactose. Gut bacteria convert the lactose to gas. Main symptoms are a lot of gas, loose stools, and stomach bloating. Onset usually at age 4 or 5. This most often runs in the family (genetic).

Diarrhea Scale

▸ **Mild:** 3 to 5 watery stools per day.

▸ **Moderate:** 6 to 9 watery stools per day.

▸ **Severe:** 10 or more watery stools per day.

▸ The main risk of diarrhea is dehydration.

▸ Loose or runny stools do not cause dehydration.

▸ Frequent, watery stools can cause dehydration.

Dehydration: How to Know

▸ Dehydration means the body has lost too much fluid. This can happen with vomiting or diarrhea. A weight loss of more than 3% is needed. Mild diarrhea or mild vomiting does not cause this. Neither does a small decrease in fluid intake.

▸ Dehydration is the most important complication of diarrhea. Dehydration is a reason to see your doctor right away.

▸ These are signs of dehydration.

• Decreased urine (no urine in more than 8 hours) happens early in dehydration. So does a dark yellow color. If the urine is light straw colored, your child is not dehydrated.

• Dry tongue and inside of the mouth. Dry lips are not helpful.

• Dry eyes with decreased or absent tears.

- In babies, a depressed or sunken soft spot.

- Slow blood refill test: Longer than 2 seconds. First, press on the thumbnail and make it pale. Then let go. Count the seconds it takes for the nail to turn pink again. Ask your doctor to teach you how to do this test.

- Fussy, tired out, or acting ill. If your child is alert, happy, and playful, he is not dehydrated.

- A child with severe dehydration becomes too weak to stand. He can also become very dizzy when trying to stand.

Diarrhea in Breastfed Babies: How to Tell

▶ Diarrhea in a breastfed baby is sometimes hard to tell.

▶ Normal breastfed stools are loose (often runny and seedy). Stools are yellow but can sometimes be green. The green color is from bile. Runny stools can even be bordered by a water ring. These are all normal stools.

▶ Breastfed babies often pass more than 6 stools per day. Until 2 months of age, they may pass a stool after each feeding. But, if stools suddenly increase in number and looseness, suspect diarrhea. If this lasts for 3 or more stools, your baby has diarrhea.

▶ If the stools contain mucus or blood or smell bad, this points to diarrhea.

▶ Other clues to diarrhea are poor eating, acting sick, or a fever.

Diarrhea in Formula-Fed Babies: How to Tell

▶ Formula-fed babies pass 1 to 8 stools per day during the first week. Then that starts to slow down to 1 to 4 per day. This lasts until 2 months of age.

▶ Stools are yellow in color and thick like peanut butter.

▶ Suspect diarrhea if the stools suddenly increase in number or looseness. If this lasts for 3 or more stools, your baby has diarrhea.

▶ If the stools contain mucus or blood or smell bad, this points to diarrhea.

▶ Other clues to diarrhea are poor eating, acting sick, or a fever.

▶ After 2 months of age, most babies pass 1 or 2 stools per day. They can also pass 1 every other day. They no longer appear to have mild diarrhea.

When to Call Your Doctor

Call 911 Now (Your Child May Need an Ambulance) If

▸ Not moving.

▸ Too weak or dizzy to stand.

▸ You think your child has a life-threatening emergency.

Call Your Doctor Now (Night or Day) If

▸ Dehydration suspected (no urine in more than 8 hours, dark urine, very dry mouth, and no tears).

▸ Blood in the stool.

▸ Constant stomach pain lasts more than 2 hours.

▸ Vomits clear liquids 3 or more times.

▸ **Age:** Younger than 1 month with 3 or more diarrhea stools in the past 24 hours.

▸ Severe diarrhea (10 or more watery stools in the last 24 hours).

▸ Fever above 104°F (40°C).

▸ **Age:** Younger than 12 weeks with fever. (**Caution:** Do *not* give your baby any fever medicine before being seen.)

▸ Weak immune system (such as sickle cell disease, HIV, cancer, organ transplant, or taking oral steroids).

▸ Your child looks or acts very sick.

▸ You think your child needs to be seen, and the problem is urgent.

Call Your Doctor Within 24 Hours If

▸ Moderate diarrhea (6 or more watery stools in the last 24 hours).

▸ Stomach pains do not go away after each diarrhea stool.

▸ Loss of bowel control in a toilet-trained child occurs 3 or more times.

▸ Fever lasts more than 3 days.

▸ Close contact with person or animal who has bacterial diarrhea.

▸ Contact with reptile (snake, lizard, or turtle) in past 14 days.

▸ Travel to country at risk for diarrhea within past month.

▸ You think your child needs to be seen, but the problem is not urgent.

Call Your Doctor During Weekday Office Hours If

▶ Diarrhea lasts more than 2 weeks.

▶ Loose stools are a frequent problem.

▶ You have other questions or concerns.

Parent Care at Home If

▶ Mild diarrhea (probably caused by a virus).

Care Advice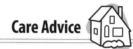

Treatment for Mild Diarrhea

❶ What You Should Know About Diarrhea

■ Most diarrhea is caused by a virus.

■ Bacterial infections as a cause of diarrhea are not common.

■ Diarrhea is the body's way of getting rid of germs.

■ The main risk of diarrhea is dehydration. Dehydration means the body has lost too much fluid.

■ Most children with diarrhea don't need to see their doctor.

■ **Note:** One or 2 loose stools can be normal with changes in diet. Diarrheal illness means 3 or more watery stools per day.

■ Here are some tips on how to keep ahead of the fluid losses.

❷ Mild Diarrhea

■ Most kids with diarrhea can eat a normal diet.

■ Drink more fluids to prevent dehydration. Formula, breast milk, or regular milk are good choices for diarrhea.

■ Do not use fruit juices or full-strength sports drinks. (**Reason:** They can make diarrhea worse.)

■ **Solid foods:** Eat more starchy foods (such as cereal, crackers, rice, or pasta). (**Reason:** They are easy to digest.)

❸ Formula-Fed Babies With Frequent, Watery Diarrhea

■ Keep giving formula but feed more often. Offer as much formula as your baby will take.

- Mix formula the normal way. (**Reason:** Formula contains plenty of water and doesn't need more.)

- **Solid foods:** If on baby foods, continue them. Cereals are best.

❹ Breastfed Babies With Frequent, Watery Diarrhea

- Give your baby breast milk more often.

- Also, give some extra fluid if breast milk isn't keeping up with fluid losses. You can use formula or oral rehydration solution (ORS) (such as Pedialyte).

- **Solid foods:** If on baby foods, continue them. Cereals are best.

❺ Older Children (Age: Older Than 1 Year) With Frequent, Watery Diarrhea

- Offer as much fluid as your child will drink. If he is also eating solid foods, water is fine. So is half-strength Gatorade or half-strength apple juice.

- If he won't eat solid foods, give milk or formula as the fluid.

- **Caution:** Do not use most fruit juices, full-strength sports drinks, or soft drinks. (**Reason:** They can make diarrhea worse.)

- **Solid foods:** Starchy foods are easy to digest and are best. Offer cereals, bread, crackers, rice, pasta, or mashed potatoes. Pretzels or salty crackers will help add some salt to meals. Some salt is good.

❻ Oral Rehydration Solutions Such as Pedialyte

- Oral rehydration solution is a special fluid that can help your child stay hydrated. You can use Pedialyte or the store brand. It can be bought in food stores or drugstores.

- **When to use:** Start ORS for frequent, watery diarrhea if you think your child is getting dehydrated. That means passing less urine than normal. Also, continue giving breast milk, formula, or regular milk.

- **Amount:** For babies, give 2 to 4 ounces (60–120 mL) of ORS after every large, watery stool.

- For children older than 1 year, give 4 to 8 ounces (120–240 mL) of ORS after every large, watery stool. Children rarely need ORS after age 3.

- **Caution:** Do not give ORS as the only fluid for more than 6 hours. (**Reason:** Your child will need calories and cry in hunger.)

❼ Probiotics

- Probiotics are healthy bacteria (such as lactobacilli). They can replace harmful bacteria in the gut (stomach).

- Probiotics may be helpful in reducing the number of diarrhea stools.

- **Age:** Older than 12 months. Yogurt is the easiest source of probiotics. Give 2 to 6 ounces (60–180 mL) of yogurt. Do this twice daily. (**Note:** Today, almost all yogurts are "active culture.")

- Probiotic supplements can also be bought in health food stores.

❽ Fever Medicine

- For fevers above 102°F (39°C), give an acetaminophen product (such as Tylenol).

- Another choice is an ibuprofen product (such as Advil).

- **Note:** Fevers under 102°F (39°C) are important for fighting infections.

- **For all fevers:** Keep your child well hydrated. Give lots of cold fluids.

❾ Diaper Rash: Prevention

- Wash buttocks after each stool to prevent a bad diaper rash.

- To protect the skin, use an ointment (such as Vaseline or Desitin). Put it on the skin around the anus.

❿ Return to School

- Your child can go back to school after stools are formed.

- The fever should also be gone.

- An older child can go back if the diarrhea is mild.

- A toilet-trained child also needs to have good control over loose stools.

⓫ What to Expect

- Viral diarrhea lasts 5 to 14 days.

- Severe diarrhea occurs only on the first or second day. But, loose stools can last for 1 to 2 weeks.

⓬ Call Your Doctor If

- Blood in the diarrhea.

- Dehydration suspected (no urine in more than 8 hours, dark urine, very dry mouth, and no tears).

- Diarrhea lasts more than 2 weeks.

- You think your child needs to be seen.

- Your child becomes worse.

Preventing Diarrhea Disease

❶ Safety Tips in All Countries

- Hand washing is the key to preventing spread of infections.
- Always wash the hands before eating, feeding, or handling young children or cooking.
- Always wash the hands after any contact with vomit or stools.
- Wash the hands after using the toilet or changing diapers. Help young children wash their hands after using the toilet.
- Fully cook all poultry. Never serve chicken that is still pink inside. (**Reason:** Undercooked poultry is a common cause of diarrhea in developed countries.)

❷ Extra Safety Tips in Developing Countries

- Drink bottled or boiled water. Avoid tap water, ice cubes, and flavored ices.
- Eat foods that have been fully cooked and are still hot.
- Dry foods such as bread are usually safe.
- Avoid salads and raw vegetables. Avoid fruits that cannot be peeled. Bananas, oranges, and apples are safe. Wash your hands before peeling fruit.
- Avoid all undercooked meat and fish.
- Avoid buying foods and drinks from street vendors. (**Reason:** This is a common cause of traveler's diarrhea.)
- Formula for babies: Breastfeed if possible. If not, use premixed formula. If you prepare your own, mix the formula with bottled or boiled water.
- Feeding babies: Wash bottles, nipples, spoons, and dishes with soap and water. Then sterilize them in boiling water for 5 minutes if possible.
- Brush your teeth with bottled or boiled water.

❸ Call Your Doctor If

- You have other questions or concerns.

Remember!
Contact your doctor if your child develops any of
the **Call Your Doctor** symptoms.

CHAPTER 35

Vomiting With Diarrhea

Definition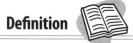

- ▶ Vomiting and diarrhea occur together. **Exception:** If vomiting is done, see Chapter 34, Diarrhea.

- ▶ Vomiting is the forceful emptying (throwing up) of what is in the stomach.

- ▶ It's normal for nausea (upset stomach) to come before each bout of vomiting.

See Other Chapter If

- ▶ Vomiting without diarrhea (Chapter 36).

- ▶ Diarrhea (Chapter 34) is the main symptom (vomiting is gone).

Causes of Vomiting With Diarrhea

- ▶ **Viral gastroenteritis.** Gastrointestinal infection from a virus is the most common cause. A common agent is the *Rotavirus*. The illness starts with vomiting. Watery, loose stools follow within 12 to 24 hours. On cruise ship outbreaks, the most common viral cause is *Norovirus*.

- ▶ **Food poisoning.** This causes rapid vomiting and diarrhea within hours after eating the bad food. Caused by toxins from germs growing in foods left out too long. An example is staph toxin in egg salad.

- ▶ **Traveler's diarrhea.** Caused by germs in food or drink. Suspect this if it follows recent foreign travel.

- ▶ **Bacterial gastrointestinal infection.** Diarrhea can also be caused by some bacteria. Most bacterial diarrhea goes away on its own. A few types can cause a severe, large bowel infection (such as *Shigella* colitis).

- ▶ **Serious complication: dehydration.** This is the health problem for which the body has lost too much fluid. (See this chapter's Dehydration: How to Know section for more information.)

Vomiting Scale

- ▶ **Mild:** 1 to 2 times per day.

- ▶ **Moderate:** 3 to 7 times per day.

▸ **Severe:** Vomits everything, nearly everything, or 8 or more times per day.

▸ Severity relates even more to how long the vomiting lasts. At the start of the illness, it's common to vomit everything. This can last for 3 or 4 hours. Children often then become stable and change to mild vomiting.

▸ The main risk of vomiting is dehydration. Dehydration means the body has lost too much fluid.

▸ Watery stools with vomiting carry the greatest risk for causing dehydration.

▸ The younger the child, the greater the risk for dehydration.

Diarrhea Scale

▸ **Mild:** 3 to 5 watery stools per day.

▸ **Moderate:** 6 to 10 watery stools per day.

▸ **Severe:** More than 10 watery stools per day.

▸ The main risk of diarrhea is dehydration.

▸ Frequent, watery stools can cause dehydration.

▸ Loose or runny stools do not cause dehydration.

Dehydration: How to Know

▸ Dehydration means the body has lost too much fluid. This can happen with vomiting or diarrhea. A weight loss of more than 3% is needed. Mild diarrhea or mild vomiting does not cause this. Neither does a small decrease in fluid intake.

▸ Vomiting with watery diarrhea is the most common cause of dehydration.

▸ Dehydration is a reason to see a doctor right away.

▸ These are signs of dehydration.

• Decreased urine (no urine in more than 8 hours) happens early in dehydration. So does a dark yellow color. If the urine is light straw colored, your child is not dehydrated.

• Dry tongue and inside of the mouth. Dry lips are not helpful.

• Dry eyes with decreased or absent tears.

• In babies, a sunken soft spot.

• Slow blood refill test: Longer than 2 seconds. First, press on the thumbnail and make it pale. Then let go. Count the seconds it takes for the nail to turn pink again. Ask your doctor to teach you how to do this test.

- Fussy, tired out, or acting ill. If your child is alert, happy, and playful, she is not dehydrated.

- A child with severe dehydration becomes too weak to stand. She can also become very dizzy when trying to stand.

When to Call Your Doctor

Call 911 Now (Your Child May Need an Ambulance) If

▸ Can't wake up.

▸ Not moving or too weak to stand.

▸ You think your child has a life-threatening emergency.

Go to ER Now If

▸ Hard to wake up.

▸ Acts or talks confused.

▸ Not alert when awake (out of it).

▸ Blood in the vomit that's not from a nosebleed.

▸ Bile (green color) in the vomit. (**Exception:** Stomach juice that is yellow.)

▸ Appendicitis suspected (pain low on right side, won't jump, wants to lie still).

▸ Poisoning suspected.

Call Your Doctor Now (Night or Day) If

▸ Dehydration suspected (no urine in more than 8 hours, dark urine, very dry mouth, and no tears).

▸ Blood in the stool.

▸ Stomach pain when not vomiting. (**Exception:** Stomach pain or crying just before vomiting is quite common.)

▸ **Age:** Younger than 12 weeks with vomiting 2 or more times. (**Exception:** Normal spitting up.)

▸ **Age:** Younger than 12 months and vomited Pedialyte 3 or more times.

▸ Severe vomiting (vomits everything) for more than 8 hours while only getting clear fluids.

▸ Weak immune system (such as sickle cell disease, HIV, cancer, organ transplant, or taking oral steroids).

▸ Vomiting a prescription medicine.

► Fever above 104°F (40°C).

► **Age:** Younger than 12 weeks with fever. (**Caution:** Do *not* give your baby any fever medicine before being seen.)

► Your child looks or acts very sick.

► You think your child needs to be seen, and the problem is urgent.

Call Your Doctor Within 24 Hours If

► **Age:** Younger than 1 year with vomiting.

► Has vomited for more than 24 hours.

► Fever lasts more than 3 days.

► You think your child needs to be seen, but the problem is not urgent.

Call Your Doctor During Weekday Office Hours If

► Vomiting is a frequent problem.

► You have other questions or concerns.

Parent Care at Home If

► Mild or moderate vomiting with diarrhea.

Care Advice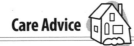

❶ What You Should Know About Vomiting With Diarrhea

■ Most vomiting is caused by a viral infection of the stomach. Sometimes, mild food poisoning is the cause.

■ Throwing up is the body's way of protecting the lower intestines.

■ Diarrhea is the body's way of getting rid of germs.

■ When vomiting and diarrhea occur together, treat the vomiting. Don't do anything special for the diarrhea.

■ The main risk of vomiting is dehydration. Dehydration means the body has lost too much fluid.

■ Here is some care advice that should help.

❷ Formula-Fed Babies: Give Oral Rehydration Solution (ORS) for 8 Hours

■ If vomits once, give half the regular amount every 1 to 2 hours.

■ If your baby vomits more than once, offer ORS for 8 hours. If you don't have ORS, use formula until you can get some.

- Oral rehydration solution is a special fluid that can help your child stay hydrated. You can use Pedialyte or the store brand of ORS. It can be bought in food stores or drugstores.

- Spoon or syringe feed small amounts. Give 1 to 2 teaspoons (5–10 mL) every 5 minutes.

- After 4 hours without your child throwing up, double the amount.

- **Return to formula.** After 8 hours without your child throwing up, go back to regular formula.

❸ Breastfed Babies: Reduce the Amount per Feeding

- If vomits once, nurse half the regular time every 1 to 2 hours.

- If your baby vomits more than once, breastfeed for 5 minutes every 30 to 60 minutes. After 4 hours without your child throwing up, return to regular breastfeeding.

- If she continues to vomit, switch to pumped breast milk. (ORS, such as Pedialyte, is rarely needed in breastfed babies. It can be used if vomiting becomes worse.)

- Spoon or syringe feed small amounts of pumped breast milk. Give 1 to 2 teaspoons (5–10 mL) every 5 minutes.

- After 4 hours without your child throwing up, return to regular feeding at the breast. Start with small feedings of 5 minutes every 30 minutes. As your baby keeps down smaller amounts, slowly give more.

❹ Children Older Than 1 Year: Offer Small Amounts of Oral Rehydration Solution for 8 Hours

- Vomiting with watery diarrhea needs ORS (such as Pedialyte). If your child refuses ORS, use a half-strength sports drink (such as Gatorade). Make it by mixing equal amounts of Gatorade and water.

- The key to success is giving small amounts of fluid. Offer 2 to 3 teaspoons (10–15 mL) every 5 minutes. Older kids can just slowly sip ORS.

- After 4 hours without your child throwing up, increase the amount.

- After 8 hours without your child throwing up, go back to regular fluids.

- Avoid fruit juices and soft drinks. They make diarrhea worse.

❺ Stop All Solid Foods

- Avoid all solid foods and baby foods in kids who are vomiting.

- After 8 hours without your child throwing up, gradually add them back.

- Start with starchy foods that are easy to digest. Examples are cereals, crackers, and bread.

❻ Do Not Give Medicines

- Stop using any drug that is over-the-counter for 8 hours. (**Reason:** Some of these can make vomiting worse.)
- **Fever:** Mild fevers don't need to be treated with any drugs. For higher fevers, you can use an acetaminophen suppository (such as FeverAll). This is a form of the drug you put in the rectum (bottom). Ask a pharmacist for help finding this product. Do not use ibuprofen. It can upset the stomach.
- **Call your doctor if** your child vomits a drug ordered by your doctor.

❼ Return to School

- Your child can return to school after the vomiting and fever are gone.

❽ What to Expect

- For the first 3 or 4 hours, your child may vomit everything. Then the stomach settles down.
- Moderate vomiting usually stops within 12 to 24 hours.
- Mild vomiting (1–2 times per day) with diarrhea may last a little longer. It can continue off and on for up to a week.

❾ Call Your Doctor If

- Vomits all clear fluids for more than 8 hours.
- Vomiting lasts more than 24 hours.
- Blood or bile (green color) in the vomit.
- Stomach pain present even when not vomiting.
- Dehydration suspected (no urine in more than 8 hours, dark urine, very dry mouth, and no tears).
- Diarrhea becomes severe.
- You think your child needs to be seen.
- Your child becomes worse.

Remember!
Contact your doctor if your child develops any of the **Call Your Doctor** symptoms.

CHAPTER 36

Vomiting Without Diarrhea

Definition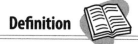

- ► Vomiting (throwing up) of stomach contents.
- ► It's normal for nausea (upset stomach) to come before each bout of vomiting.

See Other Chapter If

- ► Vomits and has diarrhea (3 or more watery or very loose stools). See Chapter 35, Vomiting With Diarrhea.
- ► Vomits only while coughing. See Chapter 26, Cough.
- ► Diarrhea is the main symptom. See Chapter 34, Diarrhea.

Causes of Vomiting

- ► **Viral gastritis.** Stomach infection from a stomach virus is the most common cause. Also called *stomach flu*. A common cause is the *Rotavirus*. The illness starts with vomiting. Watery loose stools may follow within 12 to 24 hours.
- ► **Food poisoning.** This causes rapid vomiting within hours after eating the bad food. Diarrhea may follow. Caused by toxins from germs growing in foods left out too long. An example is staph toxin in egg salad.
- ► **Ibuprofen.** Ibuprofen products (such as Advil) can be a stomach irritant. If taken on an empty stomach, they can cause vomiting.
- ► **Food allergy.** Vomiting can be a symptom of a food reaction. The vomiting comes on quickly after eating the food. Common foods are peanuts, tree nuts, fish, and shellfish (such as shrimp).
- ► **Coughing.** Hard coughing can also cause your child to throw up. This is more common in children with reflux.
- ► **Motion sickness.** Vomiting and dizziness are triggered by motion. Sea sickness or fun-park ride sickness are the most common types. Strongly genetic.
- ► **Migraines.** In children, most migraines also lead to vomiting.

- **Serious causes.** Vomiting alone (without diarrhea) should stop within 24 hours. If it lasts more than 24 hours, you must think about more serious causes. Examples are appendicitis, a kidney infection, diabetes, and head injury. A serious cause in young babies is pyloric stenosis. See this chapter's Pyloric Stenosis (Serious Cause) section for more information.

- **Cyclic vomiting.** Cyclic vomiting is the most common cause of recurrent attacks of vomiting. Attacks have a sudden onset and offset. Often occur in children who later develop migraines.

Pyloric Stenosis (Serious Cause)

- The most common cause of true vomiting in young babies.

- Onset of vomiting is age 2 weeks to 2 months.

- Vomiting is forceful. It becomes projectile and shoots out.

- Right after vomiting, the baby is hungry and wants to feed ("hungry vomiter").

- **Cause:** The pylorus is the channel between the stomach and gut. In these babies, it becomes narrow and tight.

- **Risk:** Weight loss or dehydration.

- **Treatment:** Cured by surgery.

Vomiting Scale

- **Mild:** 1 to 2 times per day.

- **Moderate:** 3 to 7 times per day.

- **Severe:** Vomits everything, nearly everything, or 8 or more times per day.

- Severity relates even more to how long the vomiting lasts. At the start of illness, it's common for a child to vomit everything. This can last for 3 or 4 hours. Children often then become stable and change to mild vomiting.

- The main risk of vomiting is dehydration. Dehydration means the body has lost too much fluid.

- The younger the child, the greater the risk for dehydration.

Dehydration: How to Tell

- The main risk of vomiting is dehydration. Dehydration means the body has lost too much water.

- Vomiting with watery diarrhea is the most common cause of dehydration.

- Dehydration is a reason to see a doctor right away.

▶ Your child may be dehydrated if

• Not drinking much fluid.

• Urine is dark yellow and has not passed in more than 8 hours.

• Inside the mouth and tongue are very dry.

• There are no tears if your child cries.

• Slow blood refill test: Longer than 2 seconds. First, gently press on the thumbnail and make it pale. Then let go. Count the seconds it takes for the nail to turn pink again. Check with your doctor if you need assistance on how to do this.

• A child with severe dehydration becomes too weak to stand or becomes very dizzy when trying to stand.

When to Call Your Doctor

Call 911 Now (Your Child May Need an Ambulance) If

▶ Can't wake up.

▶ Not moving or too weak to stand.

▶ You think your child has a life-threatening emergency.

Go to ER Now If

▶ Hard to wake up.

▶ Acts or talks confused.

▶ Not alert when awake (out of it).

▶ Stiff neck (can't touch chin to chest).

▶ Blood in the vomit that's not from a nosebleed.

▶ Bile (green color) in the vomit. (**Exception:** Stomach juice that is yellow.)

▶ Appendicitis suspected (pain low on right side, won't jump, wants to lie still).

▶ Poisoning suspected.

▶ Swallowed object suspected (such as a coin).

Call Your Doctor Now (Night or Day) If

▶ Dehydration suspected (no urine in more than 8 hours, dark urine, very dry mouth, and no tears).

- Stomach pain when not vomiting. (**Exception:** Stomach pain or crying just before vomiting is quite common.)
- Severe headache.
- Diabetes suspected (drinking lots, frequent urine, or weight loss).
- Kidney infection suspected (side or back pain, fever, or painful to pass urine).
- **Age:** Younger than 12 weeks with vomiting 2 or more times. (**Exception:** Normal spitting up.)
- Severe vomiting (vomiting everything) for more than 8 hours while getting clear fluids.
- High-risk child (such as with diabetes, or stomach or head injury).
- Weak immune system (such as sickle cell disease, HIV, cancer, organ transplant, or taking oral steroids).
- Vomiting a prescription medicine.
- Fever above 104°F (40°C).
- **Age:** Younger than 12 weeks with fever. (**Caution:** Do *not* give your baby any fever medicine before being seen.)
- Your child looks or acts very sick.
- You think your child needs to be seen, and the problem is urgent.

Call Your Doctor Within 24 Hours If

- **Age:** Younger than 1 year with vomiting.
- Vomits for more than 24 hours.
- Fever lasts more than 3 days.
- Fever returns after being gone for more than 24 hours.
- You think your child needs to be seen, but the problem is not urgent.

Call Your Doctor During Weekday Office Hours If

- Vomiting is a frequent problem.
- You have other questions or concerns.

Parent Care at Home If

- Mild or moderate vomiting (most likely viral gastritis).

Care Advice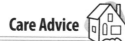

❶ What You Should Know About Vomiting Without Diarrhea

- Most vomiting is caused by a viral infection of the stomach. Sometimes, mild food poisoning is the cause.

- Vomiting is the body's way of protecting the lower gut.

- The good news is that stomach illnesses last only a short time.

- The main risk of vomiting is dehydration. Dehydration means the body has lost too much fluid.

- Here is some care advice that should help.

❷ Formula-Fed Babies: Give Oral Rehydration Solution (ORS) for 8 Hours

- If vomits once, give half the regular amount every 1 to 2 hours.

- If your baby vomits more than once, offer ORS for 8 hours. If you don't have ORS, use formula until you can get some.

- Oral rehydration solution is a special fluid that can help your child stay hydrated. You can use Pedialyte or the store brand of ORS. It can be bought in food stores or drugstores.

- Spoon or syringe feed small amounts. Give 1 to 2 teaspoons (5–10 mL) every 5 minutes.

- After 4 hours without your child throwing up, double the amount.

- **Return to formula.** After 8 hours without your child throwing up, go back to regular formula.

❸ Breastfed Babies: Reduce the Amount per Feeding

- If vomits once, nurse half the regular time every 1 to 2 hours.

- If your baby vomits more than once, breastfeed for 5 minutes every 30 to 60 minutes. After 4 hours without your child throwing up, return to regular breastfeeding.

- If he continues to vomit, switch to pumped breast milk. (ORS, such as Pedialyte, is rarely needed in breastfed babies. It can be used if vomiting becomes worse.)

- Spoon or syringe feed small amounts of pumped breast milk. Give 1 to 2 teaspoons (5–10 mL) every 5 minutes.

■ After 4 hours without your child throwing up, return to regular feeding at the breast. Start with small feedings of 5 minutes every 30 minutes. As your baby keeps down smaller amounts, slowly give more.

❹ Children Older Than 1 Year: Offer Small Amounts of Clear Fluids for 8 Hours

■ Water or ice chips are best for older children. (**Reason:** Water is easily absorbed in the stomach.)

■ Other clear fluids: Use a half-strength sports drink (such as Gatorade). Make it by mixing equal amounts of sports drink and water. Can mix apple juice the same way. Oral rehydration solution (such as Pedialyte) is usually not needed in older children. Popsicles work great for some kids.

■ The key to success is giving small amounts of fluid. Offer 2 to 3 teaspoons (10–15 mL) every 5 minutes. Older kids can slowly sip a clear fluid.

■ After 4 hours without your child throwing up, increase the amount.

■ After 8 hours without your child throwing up, return to regular fluids.

■ **Caution:** If your child vomits for more than 12 hours, switch to ORS or half-strength sports drink.

❺ Stop All Solid Foods

■ Avoid all solid and baby foods in kids who are vomiting.

■ After 8 hours without your child throwing up, gradually add them back.

■ Start with starchy foods that are easy to digest. Examples are cereals, crackers, and bread.

❻ Do Not Give Medicines

■ Stop using any drug that is over-the-counter for 8 hours. (**Reason:** Some of these can make vomiting worse.)

■ **Fever.** Mild fevers don't need to be treated with any drugs. For higher fevers, you can use an acetaminophen suppository (such as FeverAll). This is a form of the drug you put in the rectum (bottom). Ask a pharmacist for help finding this product. Do not use ibuprofen. It can upset the stomach.

■ **Call your doctor if** your child vomits a drug ordered by your doctor.

❼ Try to Sleep

■ Help your child go to sleep for a few hours.

■ **Reason:** Sleep often empties the stomach and removes the need to vomit.

■ Your child doesn't have to drink anything if his stomach feels upset and he doesn't have any diarrhea.

❽ Return to School

- Your child can return to school or child care after the vomiting and fever are gone.

❾ What to Expect

- For the first 3 or 4 hours, your child may vomit everything. Then the stomach settles down.

- Vomiting from a viral illness often stops within 12 to 24 hours.

- Mild vomiting and nausea may last up to 3 days.

❿ Call Your Doctor If

- Vomits clear fluids for more than 8 hours.

- Vomiting lasts more than 24 hours.

- Blood or bile (green color) in the vomit.

- Stomach pain present even when not vomiting.

- Dehydration suspected (no urine in more than 8 hours, dark urine, very dry mouth, and no tears).

- You think your child needs to be seen.

- Your child becomes worse.

Remember!
Contact your doctor if your child develops any of the **Call Your Doctor** symptoms.

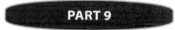

PART 9

Genital or Urinary Symptoms

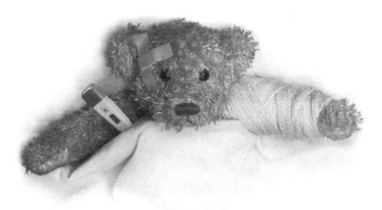

CHAPTER 37

Urination Pain

Definition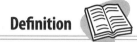

- ► Pain, burning, or stinging when a child passes urine.
- ► Also, suspect pain if your young child starts to cry while passing urine.
- ► The feeling of "can't wait" to pass urine may occur. This is called *urgency*.
- ► Passing urine more often than normal. This is called *frequency*.
- ► Pain not caused by an injury to the genitals.

Causes of Pain Passing Urine in Girls

- ► **Soap vulvitis.** Bubble bath, shampoo, or soap in bathwater is the main cause in young girls. Can cause the genital area to become red and sore. This is called *soap vulvitis*. It can cause pain when passing urine. Using a soapy washcloth can also be the cause. Vaginal itching or redness may occur. If bathing habits are not changed, it can turn into a bladder infection.
- ► **Bladder or kidney infections** (urinary tract infections) are possible at any age. They can be diagnosed by checking a urine sample.
- ► **Labial fusion** (also called *labial adhesions*). This is when the vaginal lips or folds are stuck together. The vaginal opening looks closed off. Labia that are closed more than halfway can collect soap or stool. The main symptom is itching in this area. It can also cause pain when passing urine.

Causes of Pain Passing Urine in Boys

- ► Any boy who has pain when passing urine needs his urine checked. Sometimes in young boys, the urine is normal.
- ► **Meatitis.** This means redness at the opening of the penis. It may have a sore or scab on it. Passing urine is painful. It occurs in boys who are circumcised. Can be caused by any irritant, such as bubble bath. Sometimes, the opening becomes infected with a bacteria, such as *Strep*.

▸ **Foreskin infection.** This means an infection under the foreskin. The main symptom is a red and tender foreskin. Pus may also ooze out of the foreskin opening. Passing urine is painful. It occurs in boys who are not circumcised.

▸ **Bladder or kidney infection.** Urinary tract infections are possible at any age. They are not common in boys.

When to Call Your Doctor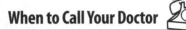

Call 911 Now (Your Child May Need an Ambulance) If

▸ Not moving or too weak to stand.

▸ You think your child has a life-threatening emergency.

Go to ER Now If

▸ Can't pass urine or can only pass a few drops.

Call Your Doctor Now (Night or Day) If

▸ Blood in urine.

▸ Severe pain when passing urine.

▸ Fever is present.

▸ Stomach, side, or back pain.

▸ Your child looks or acts very sick.

▸ You think your child needs to be seen, and the problem is urgent.

Call Your Doctor Within 24 Hours If

▸ **All boys:** Painful to pass urine but none of the symptoms above. (**Reason:** Could be a bladder infection.)

▸ **Most girls:** Painful to pass urine but none of the previously listed symptoms present. (**Reason:** Could be a bladder infection.) **Exception:** Itching or mild pain and bathes in soapy water.

Parent Care at Home If

▸ Soap vulvitis in young girl is suspected as cause.

Care Advice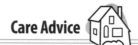

❶ What You Should Know About Soap Vulvitis in Girls

- In young girls, soap is the most common cause of pain with passing urine.
- If it does not go away within 24 hours, your child needs to have her urine checked.
- Here is some care advice that should help.

❷ Baking Soda Baths: Young Girls Only

- Soak for 10 minutes to remove germs and help with healing.
- Add 2 ounces (60 mL) baking soda per tub of warm water.
- **Reason:** Baking soda is better than vinegar for young girls.
- During soaks, be sure she spreads her legs. This allows the water to cleanse the genitals.
- Repeat baking soda soaks 2 times per day for 2 days.

❸ Do Not Use Soaps: Young Girls Only

- Do not use bubble bath, soap, and shampoo in bathwater. They can cause the genitals to be red, sore, or itchy. This is the most common cause of pain with passing urine in young girls.
- Use only warm water to cleanse the genitals.
- Baby oil can be used to remove any dried body fluids.
- After puberty, soap can be used.

❹ Vinegar Warm Water Soaks: Girls After Puberty

- Soak the genital area for 10 minutes to remove germs and irritants.
- Add 2 ounces (60 mL) vinegar per tub of warm water.
- **Reason:** After puberty, vinegar water matches normal acidity of the vagina.
- During soaks, be sure she spreads her legs. (**Reason:** This allows the water to cleanse the genital area.)
- Repeat vinegar water soaks once per day until seen by a doctor.

❺ Fluids: Offer More

- Give extra fluids to drink.
- **Reason:** Dilutes the urine so it does not sting when passed.

❻ Pain Medicine

- For pain when passing urine, give a pain medicine.
- You can use an acetaminophen product (such as Tylenol).
- Another choice is an ibuprofen product (such as Advil).
- Use as needed.

❼ Return to School

- Even if your child has a bladder infection, it cannot be spread to others.
- Your child does not need to miss any school or child care.

❽ What to Expect

- If soap is the cause, pain should go away within 24 hours.
- Itching or skin redness may last 2 days.

❾ Call Your Doctor If

- Pain when passing urine doesn't go away in 24 hours.
- Fever occurs.
- You think your child needs to be seen.
- Your child becomes worse.

Remember!
Contact your doctor if your child develops any of the **Call Your Doctor** symptoms.

CHAPTER 38

Genital Symptoms, Girls

Definition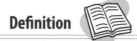

- ▶ Genital symptoms in young girls (before puberty).
- ▶ Vaginal symptoms include discharge, bleeding, and pain.
- ▶ Vaginal symptoms include itching, and pain when passing urine.
- ▶ Genital area skin symptoms include itching, pain, rash, and swelling.
- ▶ Vulva itching and irritation from soap is the most common problem.
- ▶ Symptoms not caused by an injury.

See Other Chapter If

- ▶ Pain or burning when passing urine. See Chapter 37, Urination Pain.

Causes of Genital Symptoms in Young Girls

- ▶ **Soap vulvitis.** The vulva is the area outside the vagina. Soaps can cause this area to be red, sore, and itchy. Bubble baths are the most common cause of genital itching.

- ▶ **Poor hygiene.** Not rinsing the genitals at all can also cause itching. Any stool left on the vulva is very irritating. This can happen with loose stools or back-to-front wiping. It's also seen in children who leak stool because they are blocked up. Traces of sand and dirt may do the same.

- ▶ **Yeast vulvitis.** Yeast infections of the female genital area are rare before the teen years. They do occur in girls who are still wearing diapers. They can happen after a course of antibiotics and in girls with diabetes.

- ▶ **Labial fusion** (also called *labial adhesions*). This is when the vaginal lips or folds are stuck together. The vaginal opening looks closed off. Labia that are closed more than halfway can collect soap or stool. The main symptom is itching in this area.

- ▶ **Pinworms.** Sometimes, an adult pinworm will travel into the vagina. The pinworm's secretions are very irritating. This leads to intense itching.

▸ **Vaginitis.** Vaginitis is a bacterial infection of the vagina. The main symptom is a yellow discharge. The most common cause in young girls is group A strep infection, the same one that causes bad sore throats. Vaginal discharge from sexually transmitted infections is rare before the teen years.

▸ **Vaginal foreign body (object).** Young girls may put an object (such as a bead) in the vagina. This can be part of normal behavior as young girls explore their bodies. It will cause a bad-smelling discharge. If the object is sharp, the discharge will be blood-tinged.

▸ **Bladder infection.** These are common in young girls because the urethra is so short. The main symptom is pain or burning when passing urine.

▸ **Skin rash.** Most skin rashes are from contact with some irritant. The irritant is often on dirty hands. The cause is from not washing them before using the toilet.

▸ **Serious cause: sexual abuse.** Suspect for any symptoms that are strange or not explained.

Soap Vulvitis

▸ Soap is the most common cause of genital itching in young girls. It can also cause the area to become red and sore. This is called *soap* or *chemical vulvitis.*

▸ The vulva is very sensitive to the drying effect of soaps.

▸ Sitting for a long time in a bubble bath is the main cause.

▸ Shampoo or soap in bathwater can also cause redness and itching. So can washing the genitals with a soapy washcloth.

▸ In young girls, the inner female genitals should be washed only with warm water. Skin around the genitals can be washed with soap.

▸ Soap vulvitis occurs in young girls only before puberty. Breast buds are the first sign of puberty. This diagnosis is easy if young girls are taking bubble baths.

When to Call Your Doctor

Call Your Doctor Now (Night or Day) If

▸ Could be from sexual abuse.

▸ Vaginal bleeding.

▸ Severe genital pain.

▶ Your child looks or acts very sick.

▶ You think your child needs to be seen, and the problem is urgent.

Call Your Doctor Within 24 Hours If

▶ Vaginal discharge.

▶ Fever is present.

▶ Pain or burning when passing urine.

▶ Vaginal pain.

▶ Vaginal foreign body (object) suspected.

▶ Genital area looks infected (such as spreading redness or draining sore).

▶ You think your child needs to be seen, but the problem is not urgent.

Call Your Doctor During Weekday Office Hours If

▶ Puberty has started. (**Reason:** Soap vulvitis is not the cause.)

▶ Vaginal itching lasts more than 3 days after using this chapter's Care Advice.

▶ Vaginal itching is a frequent problem.

▶ Mild rash of genital area lasts more than 3 days after using this chapter's Care Advice.

▶ You have other questions or concerns.

Parent Care at Home If

▶ Soap vulvitis suspected as cause of itching.

▶ Mild skin rash of genital area.

Care Advice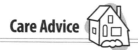

Soap Vulvitis: Treatment

❶ What You Should Know

▪ Genital itching in young girls is most often caused by soap (especially bubble baths). The vulva area is sensitive to the drying effect of soap.

▪ Clean only the genitals with warm water.

▪ After puberty, soap can be tolerated.

▪ Here is some care advice that should help.

❷ Baking Soda Baths: Young Girls Only

- Soak for 10 minutes to remove germs and help with healing.
- Add 2 ounces (60 mL) baking soda per tub of warm water.
- **Reason:** Baking soda is better than vinegar for young girls.
- During soaks, be sure she spreads her legs. This allows the water to cleanse the genitals.
- Repeat baking soda soaks 2 times per day for 2 days.

❸ Steroid Cream for Itching

- Put a tiny amount of 1% hydrocortisone cream (such as Cortaid) on the genitals.
- No prescription is needed.
- Use after soaks for 1 or 2 days. Do not use more than 2 days.

❹ Prevention: Do Not Use Soaps

- Do not use bubble bath, soap, and shampoo in bathwater. They can cause the genitals to be red, sore, or itchy.
- Use only warm water to cleanse the genitals.
- Baby oil can be used to remove any dried body fluids.
- After puberty, soap can be used.

❺ What to Expect

- If soap is the cause, symptoms should go away within 3 days.

❻ Call Your Doctor If

- Itching lasts more than 3 days after using this chapter's Care Advice.
- Vaginal discharge or bleeding occurs.
- Passing urine becomes painful.
- You think your child needs to be seen.
- Your child becomes worse.

Mild Skin Rash Near Genital Area: Treatment

❶ What You Should Know About Genital Rashes

- Rashes can be caused by skin irritants. The hand may touch the genital area when passing urine. Rashes are commonly from an irritant that was on the hands.

- Examples are a plant (such as an evergreen) or chemicals (such as bug repellents). Fiberglass, pet saliva, or even food can also be irritants.
- Most small rashes can be treated at home.
- Here is some care advice that should help.

❷ Clean the Area

- Wash the area once with soap to remove any irritants.

❸ Steroid Cream for Itching

- For itchy rashes, use 1% hydrocortisone cream (such as Cortaid). No prescription is needed.
- Do this 2 times per day for a few days.

❹ Antibiotic Ointment for Infections

- For any cuts, sores, or scabs that look infected, put on an antibiotic ointment. An example is Polysporin. No prescription is needed.
- Use 2 times per day until seen.

❺ What to Expect

- Small rashes from irritants most often go away in 3 days with treatment.

❻ Prevention of Rashes

- Teach your daughter to wash her hands if they are dirty.
- Have her clean her hands before touching her genital area.

❼ Call Your Doctor If

- Rash spreads or gets worse.
- Rash lasts more than 3 days.
- Fever occurs.
- You think your child needs to be seen.
- Your child becomes worse.

Remember!
Contact your doctor if your child develops any of
the **Call Your Doctor** symptoms.

CHAPTER 39

Genital Symptoms, Boys

Definition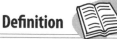

- ▶ Symptoms of the male genitals (penis or scrotum) in young boys before puberty.

- ▶ Penis symptoms include rash, pain, itching, and swelling. Discharge from the end of the penis can also occur.

- ▶ Scrotum symptoms include pain and swelling of the testicle, itching, and rash.

- ▶ Symptoms not caused by an injury.

See Other Chapter If

- ▶ Pain or burning when passing urine. See Chapter 37, Urination Pain.

Causes of Rashes on Penis or Scrotum

- ▶ Most rashes on the penis or scrotum are caused by skin irritants.

- ▶ Hand-to-penis contact is normal when passing urine. Therefore, the rash is most likely from an irritant that was on the hands.

- ▶ Examples are plants (such as weeds) or chemicals (such as bug spray). Fiberglass, pet saliva, or even food can also be irritants.

Types of Foreskin Retraction Problems

- ▶ **Paraphimosis.** Forceful retraction can cause the foreskin to get stuck behind the glans. The glans is the head of the penis. This can cause severe pain and swelling. It's a medical emergency.

- ▶ **Bleeding.** If retraction is forceful, it can cause a small cut. This cut may cause a small amount of bleeding and pain.

- ▶ **Foreskin infection.** This means an infection under the foreskin. The infection can start in a cut caused by forceful retraction. The main symptom is a red and tender foreskin. Pus may also ooze out to the foreskin opening. Passing urine is painful.

- ▶ **Urine retention (serious).** Can't pass urine or just dribbles urine, despite wanting to go.

Causes of Swollen Scrotum

▶ **Torsion of the testis (serious).** The testicle twists and cuts off its blood supply. It is always painful. Needs to be repaired within 6 to 12 hours to save the testicle. This is why seeing all males with a swollen scrotum is an emergency.

▶ **Hydrocele.** Both sides usually involved. A hydrocele is a painless sac of fluid sitting on top of the testicle. Present at birth and harmless. It goes away by a year of age.

▶ **Inguinal hernia.** A hernia is a loop of intestine that slides into the scrotum. Any new bulge that comes and goes is a hernia. All hernias need surgery to fix. Most of the time, the repair can be scheduled. If the hernia can't slide back into the abdomen, emergency surgery is needed.

▶ **Orchitis.** This is an infection of the testicle. It is always painful. It's mainly caused by virus infections, such as mumps.

When to Call Your Doctor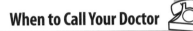

Go to ER Now If

▶ Not circumcised, and foreskin pulled back and became stuck on head of penis.

▶ Can't pass urine or can pass only a few drops.

Call Your Doctor Now (Night or Day) If

▶ Scrotum is painful or swollen.

▶ Scrotum changes to a blue or red color.

▶ Severe pain.

▶ Swollen foreskin (not circumcised).

▶ Pain or burning when passing urine, and fever.

▶ Red rash or red foreskin with fever.

▶ Could have been caused from sexual abuse.

▶ Your child looks or acts very sick.

▶ You think your child needs to be seen, and the problem is urgent.

Call Your Doctor Within 24 Hours If

▶ Pus or bloody discharge from end of penis.

▶ Pus from end of foreskin (not circumcised).

▶ Pain or burning when passing urine, but no fever.

▶ Rash is painful.

▶ Looks infected (such as draining sore or spreading redness) without fever.

▶ You think your child needs to be seen, but the problem is not urgent.

Call Your Doctor During Weekday Office Hours If

▶ Rash or itching lasts for more than 3 days after using this chapter's Care Advice.

▶ Small lump or warts.

▶ All other penis or scrotum symptoms. **Exception:** Mild rash for less than 3 days.

▶ You have other questions or concerns.

Parent Care at Home If

▶ Mild rash or itching of penis or scrotum present less than 3 days.

▶ Questions about smegma (whitish material) under the foreskin.

▶ Questions about erections in young boys.

Care Advice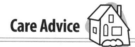

Mild Rash or Itching of Penis or Scrotum: Treatment

❶ What You Should Know About Genital Rashes

■ Rashes are more common in the summer. **Reason:** Children are outdoors and have more contact with plants and pollens. Insect bites, such as from mosquitoes or chiggers, can also be the cause.

■ Most small rashes can be treated at home.

■ Here is some care advice that should help.

❷ Clean the Area

■ Wash the area once with soap to remove any irritants.

❸ Steroid Cream for Itching

■ For itchy rashes, use 1% hydrocortisone cream (such as Cortaid). No prescription is needed.

■ Do this 2 times per day for a few days.

❹ What to Expect

- Mild rashes from irritants most often go away in 1 to 3 days with treatment.

- Severe swelling and redness may take a week to resolve.

❺ Prevention of Recurrent Symptoms

- Teach your son to wash his hands if they are dirty.

- Have him wash his hands before touching his penis.

❻ Call Your Doctor If

- Rash spreads or gets worse.

- Rash lasts more than 3 days.

- Fever occurs.

- You think your child needs to be seen.

- Your child becomes worse.

Smegma Questions

❶ Smegma: General Information

- Smegma is the small pieces of whitish material found under the foreskin. It can build up under the foreskin. This happens if the foreskin is not pulled back and cleaned regularly.

- Smegma can also occur before the foreskin becomes retractable. It lies under the foreskin that is still stuck to the head of the penis. It can't be removed.

- Smegma is made up of dead skin cells. These cells are shed from the lining of the foreskin and the penis. It becomes trapped under the foreskin.

- Smegma is normal and harmless. It is not a sign of an infection. It is produced in small amounts throughout life.

❷ Smegma Before Age 1 Year

- Sometimes, smegma can be seen through the foreskin. It looks like small whitish lumps.

- If it lies beyond the level of foreskin retraction, it should be left alone.

- Wait until normal separation exposes it.

- During your child's first year, do not make any attempts at foreskin retraction.

Erection Questions

❶ Normal Erections

- Erections in boys can occur at any age. They start in the newborn period.
- They tell us the nerves to the penis are working.
- In young boys, some are caused by a full bladder. Most occur without a clear reason.
- In teens, frequent erections start in puberty.
- Normal erections should not cause any pain.

❷ Call Your Doctor If

- Erection lasts over 1 hour.
- Erection becomes painful.

Remember!
Contact your doctor if your child develops any of the **Call Your Doctor** symptoms.

PART 10

Arm or Leg Symptoms

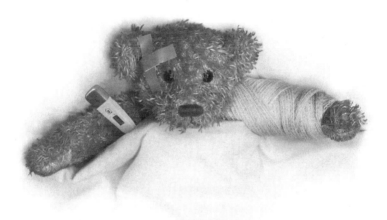

CHAPTER 40

Arm Injury

Definition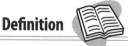

- ▶ Injuries to the arm (shoulder to fingers).
- ▶ Injuries to a bone, muscle, joint, or ligament.

See Other Chapter If

- ▶ Muscle pain caused by hard work, exercise, or sports (overuse). See Chapter 41, Arm Pain.
- ▶ Only has cuts, scrapes, or bruises. See Chapter 45, Cuts, Scrapes, and Bruises (Skin Injury).

Types of Arm Injuries

- ▶ **Fractures.** Fractures are broken bones. A broken collarbone is the most common broken bone in children. It's easy to notice because the collar bone is tender to touch. Also, the child cannot raise the arm upward.
- ▶ **Dislocations.** This happens when a bone is pulled out of a joint. A dislocated elbow is the most common type of dislocation in kids. It can happen when an adult quickly pulls or lifts a child by the arm. Mainly seen in 1- to 4-year-olds. It's also easy to spot. The arm will usually dangle straight down at the side of the body. The child is crying and unwilling to move the arm.
- ▶ **Sprains.** Sprains are stretches and tears of ligaments.
- ▶ **Strains.** Strains are stretches and tears of muscles (such as a pulled muscle).
- ▶ **Muscle overuse.** Muscle pain can occur without an injury. There is no fall or direct blow. Muscle overuse is from hard work or sports (such as a sore shoulder).
- ▶ **Muscle bruise** from a direct blow.
- ▶ **Bone bruise** from a direct blow.
- ▶ **Skin injury.** Examples are a cut, scratch, scrape, or bruise. All are common with arm injuries.

Pain Scale

▶ **Mild:** Your child feels pain and tells you about it. But, the pain does not keep your child from doing any normal activities. School, play, and sleep are not changed.

▶ **Moderate:** The pain keeps your child from doing some normal activities. It may wake your child up from sleep.

▶ **Severe:** The pain is very bad. It keeps your child from doing all normal activities.

First Aid for Bleeding

▶ Place a gauze pad or clean cloth on top of the wound.

▶ Press down firmly on the place that is bleeding.

▶ This is called *direct pressure*. It is the best way to stop bleeding.

▶ Keep using pressure until the bleeding stops.

▶ If bleeding does not stop, press on a slightly different spot.

First Aid for Suspected Fracture or Dislocation of the Shoulder

▶ Use a sling to support the arm. Create the sling with a triangular piece of cloth.

▶ Or, at the very least, your child can support the injured arm with the other hand or a pillow.

First Aid for Other Suspected Arm Fracture or Dislocation

▶ Put the arm, hand, or wrist on a hard splint so it does not move. You can use a small board, magazine folded in half, or folded-up newspaper.

▶ Tie a few cloth strips around the arm or joint to keep the splint from moving.

▶ A second choice is to use a soft splint. Wrap the arm or joint in a soft splint so it does not move. You can use a pillow, rolled-up blanket, or towel. Use tape to keep this splint in place.

▶ Put your child's injured arm in a sling. If you do not have a sling, have your child support the injured arm with his other hand.

When to Call Your Doctor

Call 911 Now (Your Child May Need an Ambulance) If

- ▶ Serious injury with many broken bones.
- ▶ Major bleeding that can't be stopped.
- ▶ Bone is sticking through the skin.
- ▶ You think your child has a life-threatening emergency.

Go to ER Now If

- ▶ Can't move the shoulder, elbow, or wrist at all.
- ▶ Looks like a broken bone (crooked or deformed).
- ▶ Looks like a dislocated joint.
- ▶ Large, deep cut that will need many stitches.

Call Your Doctor Now (Night or Day) If

- ▶ Can't move the shoulder, elbow, or wrist normally.
- ▶ Collarbone is painful, and can't raise arm over head.
- ▶ Can't open and close the hand normally.
- ▶ Skin is split open or gaping and may need stitches.
- ▶ Cut over knuckle of hand.
- ▶ **Age:** Younger than 1 year.
- ▶ Severe pain doesn't improve 2 hours after taking pain medicine.
- ▶ You think your child has a serious injury.
- ▶ You think your child needs to be seen, and the problem is urgent.

Call Your Doctor Within 24 Hours If

- ▶ Very large bruise or swelling.
- ▶ Pain not better after 3 days.
- ▶ You think your child needs to be seen, but the problem is not urgent.

Call Your Doctor During Weekday Office Hours If

▶ Injury limits sports or schoolwork.

▶ Dirty cut and no tetanus shot in more than 5 years.

▶ Clean cut and no tetanus shot in more than 10 years.

▶ Pain lasts more than 2 weeks.

▶ You have other questions or concerns.

Parent Care at Home If

▶ Bruised muscle or bone from direct blow.

▶ Pain in muscle (from minor pulled muscle).

▶ Pain around joint (from minor stretched ligament).

Care Advice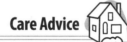

❶ What You Should Know About Minor Arm Injuries

■ During sports, muscles and bones get bruised.

■ Muscles get stretched.

■ Here is some care advice that should help.

❷ Pain Medicine

■ To help with pain, give an acetaminophen product (such as Tylenol).

■ Another choice is an ibuprofen product (such as Advil). Ibuprofen works well for this type of pain.

■ Use as needed.

❸ Cold Pack for Pain

■ For pain or swelling, use a cold pack. You can also use ice wrapped in a wet cloth.

■ Place it on the sore muscles for 20 minutes.

■ Repeat 4 times on the first day and then as needed.

■ **Reason:** Helps ease pain and stop any bleeding.

■ **Caution:** Avoid frostbite.

❹ Use Heat After 48 Hours

- If pain lasts more than 2 days, place heat on the sore muscle.
- Use a heat pack, heating pad, or warm, wet washcloth.
- Do this for 10 minutes and then as needed.
- **Reason:** Increases blood flow and improves healing.
- **Caution:** Avoid burns.

❺ Rest the Arm

- Rest the injured arm as much as possible for 48 hours.

❻ What to Expect

- Pain and swelling most often peak on day 2 or 3.
- Swelling should be gone within 7 days.
- Pain may take 2 weeks to fully go away.

❼ Call Your Doctor If

- Pain becomes severe.
- Pain is not better after 3 days.
- Pain lasts more than 2 weeks.
- You think your child needs to be seen.
- Your child becomes worse.

Remember!
Contact your doctor if your child develops any of the **Call Your Doctor** symptoms.

CHAPTER 41

Arm Pain

Definition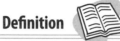

- ▶ Pain in the arm (shoulder to fingers).
- ▶ Includes shoulder, elbow, wrist, and finger joints.
- ▶ Includes minor muscle strains from hard work or sports (overuse).
- ▶ Pain not caused by an injury.

See Other Chapter If

- ▶ Arm pain after an arm injury. See Chapter 40, Arm Injury.

Causes of Arm Pain

- ▶ **Muscle overuse (strained muscles).** Arm pains are often from hard work or sports. Examples are too much throwing or swimming. They are most common in the shoulder. This type of pain can last hours up to 7 days.

- ▶ **Muscle cramps.** Brief pain that lasts 1 to 15 minutes is often due to muscle cramps. These occur in the hand after too much writing or typing.

- ▶ **Viral illness.** Mild muscle aches in both arms also occur with many viral illnesses.

- ▶ **Septic arthritis (serious).** This is a bacterial infection of a joint space. Main symptoms are fever and severe pain with movement of the joint. Range of motion is limited or absent (a "frozen joint").

Pain Scale

- ▶ **Mild:** Your child feels pain and tells you about it. The pain does not keep your child from doing any normal activities. School, play, and sleep are not changed.

- ▶ **Moderate:** The pain keeps your child from doing some normal activities. It may wake your child up from sleep.

- ▶ **Severe:** The pain is very bad. It keeps your child from doing all normal activities.

When to Call Your Doctor

Call 911 Now (Your Child May Need an Ambulance) If

▶ Not moving or too weak to stand.

▶ You think your child has a life-threatening emergency.

Call Your Doctor Now (Night or Day) If

▶ Can't use arm or hand normally.

▶ Can't move the shoulder, elbow, or wrist normally.

▶ Swollen joint.

▶ Muscles are weak (loss of strength).

▶ Numbness (loss of feeling) present more than 1 hour.

▶ Severe pain or cries when arm is touched or moved.

▶ Your child looks or acts very sick.

▶ You think your child needs to be seen, and the problem is urgent.

Call Your Doctor Within 24 Hours If

▶ Fever is present.

▶ Bright red area on skin.

▶ You think your child needs to be seen, but the problem is not urgent.

Call Your Doctor During Weekday Office Hours If

▶ Cause of arm pain is not clear.

▶ Arm pain lasts more than 7 days.

▶ Arm pains or muscle cramps are a frequent problem.

▶ You have other questions or concerns.

Parent Care at Home If

▶ Caused by overusing the muscles.

▶ Cause is clear and harmless. (Examples are a sliver that's removed or a recent shot.)

Care Advice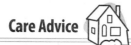

❶ What You Should Know About Mild Arm Pain

- Strained arm muscles are common after using them too much during sports.
- An example is throwing a ball over and over again.
- Weekend warriors who are out of shape get the most muscle pains.
- Here is some care advice that should help.

❷ Pain Medicine

- To help with pain, give an acetaminophen product (such as Tylenol).
- Another choice is an ibuprofen product (such as Advil).
- Use as needed.

❸ Cold Pack for Pain

- For pain or swelling, use a cold pack. You can also use ice wrapped in a wet cloth.
- Put it on the sore muscles for 20 minutes.
- Repeat 4 times on the first day and then as needed.
- **Caution:** Avoid frostbite.

❹ Use Heat After 48 Hours

- If pain lasts more than 2 days, put heat on the sore muscle.
- Use a heat pack, heating pad, or warm, wet washcloth.
- Do this for 10 minutes and then as needed.
- **Reason:** Increases blood flow and improves healing.
- **Caution:** Avoid burns.

❺ What to Expect

- A strained muscle hurts for 2 or 3 days.
- Pain often peaks on day 2.
- After severe overuse, the pain may last a week.

➏ Call Your Doctor If

- Fever or swollen joint occurs.

- Pain caused by work or sports lasts more than 7 days.

- You think your child needs to be seen.

- Pain gets worse.

Remember!
Contact your doctor if your child develops any of
the **Call Your Doctor** symptoms.

CHAPTER 42

Leg Injury

Definition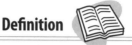

- ▶ Injuries to the leg (hip to foot).

- ▶ Injuries to a bone, muscle, joint, or ligament.

See Other Chapter If

- ▶ Muscle pain caused by too much exercise or work (overuse). See Chapter 43, Leg Pain.

- ▶ Only has cuts, scrapes, or bruises. See Chapter 45, Cuts, Scrapes, and Bruises (Skin Injury).

Types of Leg Injuries

- ▶ **Fracture.** This is the medical name for a broken bone. The most common broken bone in the leg is the tibia. The tibia is the largest bone in the lower part of the leg. Children with a fracture are not able to bear weight or walk.

- ▶ **Dislocation.** This happens when a bone is pulled out of its joint. The most common one in the leg is a dislocated kneecap (patella).

- ▶ **Sprains.** Sprains are stretches and tears of ligaments. A sprained ankle is the most common ligament injury of the leg. It's usually caused by turning the ankle inward. Also called a "twisted ankle." Main symptoms are pain and swelling of the outside of the ankle.

- ▶ **Strains.** Strains are stretches and tears of muscles (a pulled muscle).

- ▶ **Muscle overuse.** Muscle pain can occur without an injury. There is no fall or direct blow. Muscle overuse injuries are from sports or exercise. Shin splints of the lower part of the leg are often from running.

- ▶ **Muscle bruise from a direct blow.** Bleeding into the quadriceps (thigh muscles) is very painful.

- ▶ **Bone bruise from a direct blow (like on the hip).** Called a *hip pointer.*

- ▶ **Skin injury.** Examples are a cut, scratch, scrape, or bruise. All are common with leg injuries.

Pain Scale

▶ **Mild:** Your child feels pain and tells you about it. But, the pain does not keep your child from doing any normal activities. School, play, and sleep are not changed.

▶ **Moderate:** The pain keeps your child from doing some normal activities. It may wake your child up from sleep.

▶ **Severe:** The pain is very bad. It keeps your child from doing all normal activities.

First Aid for Bleeding

▶ Place a gauze pad or clean cloth on top of the wound.

▶ Press down firmly on the area that is bleeding.

▶ This is called *direct pressure*. It is the best way to stop bleeding.

▶ Keep using pressure until the bleeding stops.

▶ If bleeding does not stop, press on a slightly different spot.

First Aid for Suspected Fracture or Dislocation

▶ Put the leg or joint on a hard splint so it does not move. You can use a small board, magazine folded in half, or folded-up newspaper.

▶ Tie a few cloth strips around the leg or joint to keep the splint from moving.

▶ A second choice is to use a soft splint. Wrap the leg or joint in a soft splint so it does not move. You can use a pillow, rolled-up blanket, or towel. Use tape to keep this splint in place.

When to Call Your Doctor

Call 911 Now (Your Child May Need an Ambulance) If

▶ Major bleeding can't be stopped.

▶ Serious injury with many broken bones.

▶ Bone is sticking through the skin.

▶ Looks like a dislocated joint (hip, knee, or ankle).

▶ You think your child has a life-threatening emergency.

Go to ER Now If

▸ Looks like a broken bone (crooked or deformed).

▸ Can't stand or walk.

▸ Large, deep cut that will need many stitches.

Call Your Doctor Now (Night or Day) If

▸ Skin is split open or gaping and may need stitches.

▸ **Age:** Younger than 1 year.

▸ Severe pain doesn't improve 2 hours after taking pain medicine.

▸ Can't move hip, knee, or ankle normally.

▸ Knee injury with a "snap" or "pop" felt at the time of impact.

▸ You think your child has a serious injury.

▸ You think your child needs to be seen, and the problem is urgent.

Call Your Doctor Within 24 Hours If

▸ Has a limp when walking.

▸ Very large bruise.

▸ Large swelling.

▸ Pain not improved after 3 days.

▸ You think your child needs to be seen, but the problem is not urgent.

Call Your Doctor During Weekday Office Hours If

▸ Injury limits sports or schoolwork.

▸ Dirty cut and no tetanus shot in more than 5 years.

▸ Clean cut and no tetanus shot in more than 10 years.

▸ Pain lasts more than 2 weeks.

▸ You have other questions or concerns.

Parent Care at Home If

▸ Bruised muscle or bone from direct blow.

▸ Pain in muscle from minor pulled muscle.

▸ Pain around joint from minor stretched ligament.

Care Advice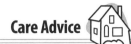

❶ What You Should Know About Minor Leg Injuries

- During sports, muscles and bones get bruised.

- Muscles get stretched.

- These injuries can be treated at home.

- Here is some care advice that should help.

❷ Pulled Muscle, Bruised Muscle, or Bruised Bone Treatment

- **Pain medicine.** To help with pain, give an acetaminophen product (such as Tylenol). Another choice is an ibuprofen product (such as Advil). Use as needed. Ibuprofen works better for this type of pain.

- **Cold pack.** For pain or swelling, use a cold pack. You can also use ice wrapped in a wet cloth. Put it on the sore muscles for 20 minutes. Repeat 4 times on the first day and then as needed. (**Reason:** Helps ease pain and stop any bleeding.) (**Caution:** Avoid frostbite.)

- **Heat pack.** If pain lasts more than 2 days, put heat on the sore muscle. Use a heat pack, heating pad, or warm, wet washcloth. Do this for 10 minutes and then as needed. (**Caution:** Avoid burns.) For stiffness allover, use a hot bath instead. Move the sore leg muscles under warm water.

- **Rest.** Rest the injured part as much as possible for 48 hours.

- **Stretching.** For pulled muscles, teach your youngster about stretching and strength training.

❸ Mild Sprains (Stretched Ligaments) of Ankle or Knee Treatment

- **First aid:** Apply ice to reduce bleeding, swelling, and pain. Wrap with an elastic bandage. The more bleeding and swelling there is, the longer it will take to get better.

- Treat with RICE (rest, ice, compression, and elevation) for the first 24 to 48 hours.

- Apply compression with a snug, elastic bandage for 48 hours. Numbness, tingling, or increased pain means the bandage is too tight.

- **Cold pack:** For pain or swelling, use a cold pack. You can also use ice wrapped in a wet cloth. Put it on the ankle or knee for 20 minutes. Repeat 4 times on the first day and then as needed. (**Reason:** Helps ease pain and stop any bleeding.) (**Caution:** Avoid frostbite.)

- To help with pain, give an acetaminophen product (such as Tylenol). Another choice is an ibuprofen product (such as Advil). Use as needed. Continue for at least 48 hours.

- Keep the injured ankle or knee elevated and at rest for 24 hours.

- After 24 hours, allow any activity that doesn't cause pain.

❹ What to Expect

- Pain and swelling usually peak on day 2 or 3.

- Most often, swelling is gone within 7 days.

- Pain may take 2 weeks to fully go away.

❺ Call Your Doctor If

- Pain becomes severe.

- Pain is not better after 3 days.

- Pain lasts more than 2 weeks.

- You think your child needs to be seen.

- Your child becomes worse.

Remember!
Contact your doctor if your child develops any of the **Call Your Doctor** symptoms.

CHAPTER 43

Leg Pain

Definition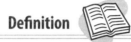

▸ Pain in the legs (hip to foot).

▸ Pain includes hip, knee, ankle, foot, and toe joints.

▸ Pain includes minor muscle strain from overuse.

▸ Muscle cramps are also covered.

▸ Pain not caused by an injury.

See Other Chapter If

▸ Leg pain after an injury. See Chapter 42, Leg Injury.

Causes

▸ **Main causes.** Muscle spasms (cramps) and strained muscles (overuse) account for most leg pain.

▸ **Muscle cramps.** Brief pains (1–15 minutes) are often due to muscle spasms (cramps). Foot or calf muscles are especially prone to cramps that occur during sports. Foot or leg cramps may also awaken your child from sleep. Muscle cramps that occur during hard work or sports are called *heat cramps*. They often respond to extra fluids and salt.

▸ **Muscle overuse (strained muscles).** Constant leg pains are often from hard work or sports. Examples are running or jumping too much. This type of pain can last several hours up to 7 days. Muscle pain can also be from a forgotten injury that occurred the day before.

▸ **Growing pains.** Ten percent of healthy children have harmless leg pains that come and go. These are often called *growing pains* (although they have nothing to do with growth). Growing pains usually occur in the calf or thigh muscles. They usually occur on both sides, not one side. They occur late in the day. Most likely, they are due to running or playing hard. They usually last 10 to 30 minutes.

▸ **Low calcium level.** Low calcium and vitamin D levels can cause low-grade bone pains. Pain is mainly in the legs and ribs. Children on a milk-free diet are at risk.

- ▸ **Osgood-Schlatter disease.** Pain, swelling, and tenderness of the bone (tibia) just below the kneecap. The patellar tendon attaches on this bone. Caused by excessive jumping or running. Peak age is the young teen years. Harmless and goes away in 1 to 2 years.

- ▸ **Viral infections.** Muscle aches in both legs are common with viral illness, especially influenza.

- ▸ **Serious causes.** Fractures, deep vein thrombosis (blood clot in leg). Also, neuritis (a nerve infection) and arthritis (a joint infection).

- ▸ **Septic arthritis (serious).** A bacterial infection of any joint space is a medical emergency. Symptoms are severe joint pain, joint stiffness, and a high fever.

- ▸ **Toxic synovitis of the hip.** It is a harmless condition. It can imitate a septic arthritis of the hip. Symptoms are a limp, moderate pain and usually no fever. Toxic synovitis tends to occur in toddlers after jumping too much.

Pain Scale

- ▸ **Mild:** Your child feels pain and tells you about it. The pain does not keep your child from doing any normal activities. School, play, and sleep are not changed.

- ▸ **Moderate:** The pain keeps your child from doing some normal activities. It may wake your child up from sleep.

- ▸ **Severe:** The pain is very bad. It keeps your child from doing all normal activities.

When to Call Your Doctor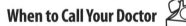

Call 911 Now (Your Child May Need an Ambulance) If

- ▸ Not moving or too weak to stand.

- ▸ You think your child has a life-threatening emergency.

Go to ER Now If

- ▸ Can't stand or walk.

Call Your Doctor Now (Night or Day) If

- ▸ Fever and pain in one leg only.

- ▸ Can't move a hip, knee, or ankle normally.

- ▸ Swollen joint.

- ▸ Calf pain on 1 side lasts more than 12 hours.

- Numbness (loss of feeling) lasts more than 1 hour.
- Severe pain or cries when leg is touched or moved.
- Your child looks or acts very sick.
- You think your child needs to be seen, and the problem is urgent.

Call Your Doctor Within 24 Hours If

- Walking is not normal (has a limp).
- Fever and pain in both legs.
- Bright red area on skin.
- You think your child needs to be seen, but the problem is not urgent.

Call Your Doctor During Weekday Office Hours If

- Cause of leg pain is not clear.
- Leg pain lasts more than 7 days.
- Leg pains or muscle cramps are a frequent problem.
- You have other questions or concerns.

Parent Care at Home If

- Muscle cramps in the calf or foot.
- Strained muscles caused by overuse (exercise or work).
- Growing pains suspected.
- Cause is clear and harmless. (Examples are tight, new shoes or a recent shot.)

Care Advice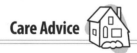

❶ What You Should Know About Leg Pain

- Strained muscles are common after too much exercise or hard sports.
- Examples are hiking or running.
- Weekend warriors who are out of shape get the most muscle pains.
- Here is some care advice that should help.

❷ Muscle Cramps Treatment

- Muscle cramps in the feet or calf muscles occur in a third of children.

- **Stretching.** During attacks, stretch the painful muscle by pulling the foot and toes upward. Stretch as far as they will go to break the spasm. Stretch in the opposite direction to how it is being pulled by the cramp.

- **Cold pack.** Use a cold pack. You can also use ice wrapped in a wet cloth. Put it on the sore muscle for 20 minutes.

- **Water.** Heat cramps can occur with hard sports on a hot day. If you suspect heat cramps, have your child drink lots of fluids. Water or sports drinks are good choices. Continue with stretching and using a cold pack.

- **Prevention.** Future attacks may be prevented by daily stretching exercises of the heel cords. Stand with the knees straight. Then, stretch the ankles by leaning forward against a wall. Place a pillow under the covers at the foot of the bed at night. This gives the feet more room to move at night. Also, be sure your child gets enough calcium in his diet. Daily vitamin D3 may also help.

❸ Strained Muscles From Overuse Treatment

- **Pain medicine.** To help with pain, give an acetaminophen product (such as Tylenol). Another choice is an ibuprofen product (such as Advil). Use as needed.

- **Cold pack.** For pain or swelling, use a cold pack. You can also use ice wrapped in a wet cloth. Put it on the sore muscles for 20 minutes. Repeat 4 times on the first day and then as needed. (**Caution:** Avoid frostbite.)

- **Heat pack.** If pain lasts more than 2 days, put heat on the sore muscle. Use a heat pack, heating pad, or warm, wet washcloth. Do this for 10 minutes and then as needed. (**Caution:** Avoid burns.) For stiffness all over, use a hot bath instead. Move the sore leg muscles under warm water.

❹ Growing Pains Treatment

- Most often, the pains are mild and don't last long. No treatment is needed.

- **Massage.** Rub the sore muscles to help the pain go away.

- **Pain medicine.** If pain lasts more than 30 minutes, give a pain medicine. You can use either acetaminophen (such as Tylenol) or ibuprofen (such as Advil). Use as needed.

- **Prevention.** Research has shown that daily stretching can prevent most growing pains. Stretch the quadriceps, hamstrings, and calf muscles.

❺ What to Expect

- Muscle cramps usually last 5 to 30 minutes.
- Once they go away, the muscle returns to normal quickly.
- A strained muscle hurts for 3 to 7 days. Pain often peaks on day 2.
- Following severe overuse, the pain may last a week.

❻ Call Your Doctor If

- Muscle cramps occur often.
- Fever, limp, or a swollen joint occurs.
- Pain caused by work or sports lasts more than 7 days.
- You think your child needs to be seen.
- Your child becomes worse.

Remember!
Contact your doctor if your child develops any of the **Call Your Doctor** symptoms.

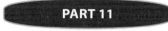

PART 11

Skin: Localized Symptoms

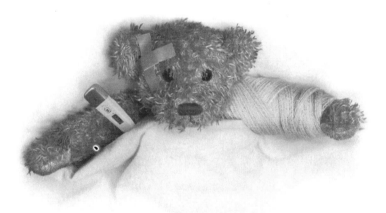

CHAPTER 44

Rash or Redness: Localized and Cause Unknown

Definition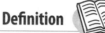

- Red or pink rash on one small part of the body (localized).
- Small spots, large spots, or solid redness.
- Includes redness from skin irritation.

See Other Chapter If
- Mosquito bite (Chapter 54).

Causes of Localized Rash or Redness
- **Irritants.** A rash in just one spot is usually caused by skin contact with an irritant.
- **Plants.** Many plants cause skin reactions. Sap from evergreens can cause a red area.
- **Pollen.** Playing in the grass can cause a pink rash on exposed skin.
- **Pet saliva.** Some people get a rash where a dog or cat has licked them.
- **Food.** Some children get a rash if a food is rubbed on the skin. An example could be a fresh fruit. Some babies get hives around the mouth from drooling while eating a new food.
- **Chemicals.** Many products used in the home can be irritating to the skin.
- **Insect bite.** Local redness and swelling is a reaction to the insect's saliva. Can be very large without being an allergy. Kids often get mosquito bites without anyone noticing it.
- **Bee sting.** Local redness and swelling is a reaction to the bee's venom. Can be very large without being an allergy.
- **Cellulitis.** This is a bacterial infection of the skin. The main symptom is a red area that keeps spreading. Starts from a break in the skin (such as a scratched insect bite). The red area is painful to the touch.

Localized Versus Widespread Rash: How to Decide

▶ *Localized* means the rash occurs on one small part of the body. Usually, the rash is just on one side of the body. An example is a rash on one foot. (**Exceptions:** Athlete's foot can occur on both feet. Insect bites can be scattered.)

▶ *Widespread* means the rash occurs on larger areas. Examples are both legs or the entire back. Widespread can also be on most of the body surface. Widespread rashes always occur on matching (both) sides of the body. Many viral rashes are on the chest, stomach, and back.

▶ Cause of a widespread rash usually goes through the bloodstream. Examples are rashes caused by viruses, bacteria, toxins, or food or drug allergies.

▶ Cause of a localized rash is usually just from contact with the skin. Examples are rashes caused by chemicals, allergens, insect bites, ringworm fungus, bacteria, or irritants.

▶ This is why it's important to make this distinction.

Contact Dermatitis

▶ Contact dermatitis is a common cause of a rash in one area. This is especially true of a small rash that will not go away. Contact dermatitis usually starts as raised, red spots. It can change to blisters, as in poison ivy. The rash is itchy. Contact dermatitis is an allergic skin rash. Location of the rash may suggest the cause.

▶ **Poison ivy or oak:** Exposed areas, such as the hands.

▶ **Nickel (metal):** Anywhere the metal has touched the skin (neck from necklaces, earlobe from earrings, fingers from rings, stomach from metal snap inside pants, wrist from watch, or face from eyeglass frames).

▶ **Tanning agents in leather:** Tops of the feet from shoes or hands from leather gloves.

▶ **Preservatives** in creams, lotions, cosmetics, sunscreens, or shampoos where applied.

▶ **Neomycin** in antibiotic ointment where applied.

When to Call Your Doctor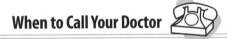

Call 911 Now (Your Child May Need an Ambulance) If

▶ Not moving or too weak to stand.

▶ You think your child has a life-threatening emergency.

Call Your Doctor Now (Night or Day) If

▶ Purple or blood-colored spots or dots that are not from injury or friction.

▶ **Age:** Younger than 1 month with tiny water blisters.

▶ Your child looks or acts very sick.

▶ You think your child needs to be seen, and the problem is urgent.

Call Your Doctor Within 24 Hours If

▶ Bright red area or red streak (but not sunburn).

▶ Rash is very painful.

▶ Fever is present.

▶ Severe itching.

▶ Looks like a boil, infected sore, or other infected rash.

▶ Teen with a rash on the genitals.

▶ Lyme disease suspected (bull's-eye rash and tick bite or contact).

▶ You think your child needs to be seen, but the problem is not urgent.

Call Your Doctor During Weekday Office Hours If

▶ Blisters without a clear cause. (**Exception:** Poison ivy.)

▶ Pimples. (Use an antibiotic ointment until seen.)

▶ Rash grouped in a stripe or band.

▶ Peeling fingers.

▶ Rash lasts more than 7 days.

▶ You have other questions or concerns.

Parent Care at Home If

▶ Mild localized rash or redness.

Care Advice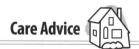

❶ What You Should Know About Localized Rashes

■ Most new localized rashes are due to skin contact with an irritating substance.

■ Here is some care advice that should help.

❷ Avoid the Cause

- Try to find the cause.

- Consider irritants like a plant (such as evergreens or weeds). Also, chemicals (such as solvents or insecticides). Irritants can also include fiberglass or detergents. A new cosmetic or jewelry (such as nickel) may also be the cause.

- A pet may carry the irritant, as with poison ivy or oak. Also, your child could react directly to pet saliva.

- Review the list of causes for this chapter's Contact Dermatitis section on page 262.

❸ Do Not Use Soap

- Wash the red area once with soap to remove any remaining irritants.

- Then, do not use soaps on it. (**Reason:** Soaps can slow healing.)

- Cleanse the area when needed with warm water.

❹ Cold Soaks for Itching

- Use a cold, wet washcloth or soak in cold water for 20 minutes.

- Do this every 3 to 4 hours as needed. This will help with itching or pain.

❺ Steroid Cream for Itching

- If the itch is more than mild, use 1% hydrocortisone cream (such as Cortaid). Put it on the rash.

- No prescription is needed.

- Use it 3 times per day.

- **Exception:** Do not use for suspected ringworm.

❻ Try Not to Scratch

- Help your child not scratch.

- Cut the fingernails short.

❼ Return to School

- Children with localized rashes do not need to miss any child care or school.

❽ What to Expect

- Most of these rashes go away in 2 to 3 days.

❾ Call Your Doctor If

- Rash spreads or gets worse.

- Rash lasts for more than 1 week.

- You think your child needs to be seen.

- Your child becomes worse.

Remember!
Contact your doctor if your child develops any of the **Call Your Doctor** symptoms.

CHAPTER 45

Cuts, Scrapes, and Bruises (Skin Injury)

Definition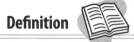

- ▶ Injuries to the skin anywhere on the body surface.
- ▶ Includes cuts, scratches, scrapes, bruises, and swelling.

See Other Chapter If

- ▶ **Animal or human bite.** See Chapter 52, Animal or Human Bite.
- ▶ **Stab wound or puncture.** See Chapter 46, Puncture Wound.
- ▶ **A sliver is in the skin.** See Chapter 47, Skin Foreign Body or Object (Splinters).
- ▶ **Injury looks infected.** See Chapter 48, Wound Infection.

Types of Skin Injury

- ▶ **Cuts, lacerations, gashes, and tears.** These are wounds that go through the skin to the fat tissue. Caused by a sharp object.

- ▶ **Scrapes, abrasions, scratches, and floor burns.** These are surface wounds that don't go all the way through the skin. Scrapes are common on the knees, elbows, and palms.

- ▶ **Bruises.** These are bleeding into the skin from damaged blood vessels. Caused by a blunt object. They can occur without a cut or scrape.

When Sutures (Stitches) Are Needed for Cuts

- ▶ Any cut that is split open or gaping needs sutures.

- ▶ Cuts longer than ½ in (1.3 cm) usually need sutures.

- ▶ On the face, cuts longer than ¼ in (6 mm) usually need to be seen. They usually need closure with sutures or skin glue.

- ▶ Any open wound that may need sutures should be seen as soon as possible. Ideally, they should be checked and closed within 6 hours. (**Reason:** To prevent wound infections.) There is no cutoff, however, for treating open wounds.

Cuts Versus Scratches: Helping You Decide

▸ The skin is about ⅛ in (3 mm) thick.

▸ A cut (laceration) goes through it.

▸ A scratch or scrape (wide scratch) doesn't go through the skin.

▸ Cuts that gape open at rest or with movement need stitches to prevent scarring.

▸ Scrapes and scratches never need stitches, no matter how long they are.

First Aid for Bleeding

▸ Place a gauze pad or clean cloth on top of the wound.

▸ Press down firmly on the place that is bleeding.

▸ This is called *direct pressure*. It is the best way to stop bleeding.

▸ Keep using pressure until the bleeding stops.

▸ If bleeding does not stop, press on a slightly different spot.

First Aid for Shock

▸ Lie down with the feet elevated.

First Aid for Penetrating Object

▸ If penetrating object still in place, don't remove it. (**Reason:** Removal can increase bleeding.)

When to Call Your Doctor

Call 911 Now (Your Child May Need an Ambulance) If

▸ Major bleeding that can't be stopped.

▸ Deep cut to chest, stomach, head, or neck (such as with a knife).

Go to ER Now If

▸ Bleeding won't stop after 10 minutes of direct pressure.

▸ Deep cut and can see bone or tendons.

▸ Large, deep cut that will need many stitches.

Call Your Doctor Now (Night or Day) If

- Skin is split open or gaping and may need stitches.

- Severe pain doesn't improve 2 hours after taking pain medicine.

- **Age:** Younger than 1 year.

- Dirt in the wound is not gone after 15 minutes of scrubbing.

- Skin loss from bad scrape goes very deep.

- Bad scrape covers large area.

- Cut or scrape looks infected (spreading redness, red streak).

- Cut or scrape and no past tetanus shots.

- You think your child has a serious injury.

- You think your child needs to be seen, and the problem is urgent.

Call Your Doctor Within 24 Hours If

- Very large bruise after a minor injury.

- Some bruises appear without any known injury.

- You think your child needs to be seen, but the problem is not urgent.

Call Your Doctor During Weekday Office Hours If

- Dirty cut and no tetanus shot in more than 5 years.

- Clean cut and no tetanus shot in more than 10 years.

- Doesn't heal by 10 days.

- You have other questions or concerns.

Parent Care at Home If

- Minor cut, scrape, or bruise (minor bleeding that stops).

Care Advice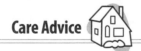

❶ Cuts, Scratches, and Scrapes: Treatment

- Use direct pressure to stop any bleeding. Do this for 10 minutes or until the bleeding stops.

- Wash the wound with soap and water for 5 minutes. Try to rinse the cut under running water.

- **Caution:** Never soak a wound that might need sutures. (**Reason:** It may become more swollen and harder to close.)

- Gently scrub out any dirt with a washcloth.

- Use an antibiotic ointment (such as Polysporin). No prescription is needed. Then, cover it with a bandage (such as a Band-Aid). Change daily.

❷ Liquid Skin Bandage for Minor Cuts

- Liquid skin bandage seals wounds with a plastic coating. It lasts up to 1 week.

- Liquid skin bandage has several benefits compared with other bandages (such as a Band-Aid). Liquid bandage needs to be put on only once. It seals the wound and may promote faster healing and lower infection rates. Also, it's waterproof.

- Use for any small break in the skin. Examples are paper cuts, hangnails, and cracks on the fingers or toes.

- Wash and dry the wound first. Then, put on the liquid. It comes with a brush or swab. It dries in less than a minute.

- You can get this product at a drugstore near you. There are many brands of liquid bandage. No prescription is needed.

❸ Bruises: Treatment

- Use a cold pack or ice bag wrapped in a wet cloth. Put it on the bruise once for 20 minutes. This will help stop the bleeding.

- After 48 hours, use a warm, wet washcloth. Do this for 10 minutes 3 times per day. This helps reabsorb the blood.

❹ Pain Medicine

- To help with pain, give an acetaminophen product (such as Tylenol).

- Another choice is an ibuprofen product (such as Advil).

- Use as needed.

❺ Tetanus Shot

- A tetanus shot update may be needed for cuts and other open wounds.

- Check your vaccine records to see when your child got the last one.

- For dirty cuts and scrapes: If last tetanus shot was given more than 5 years ago, your child will need a booster.

- For clean cuts: If last tetanus shot was given more than 10 years ago, your child will need a booster.

- See your child's doctor for a booster during regular office hours. It's safe to give it within 3 days or less.

❻ What to Expect

- Small cuts and scrapes heal in less than a week.

❼ Call Your Doctor If

- Bleeding does not stop after applying direct pressure on the cut.

- Starts to look infected (pus, redness).

- Doesn't heal within 10 days.

- You think your child needs to be seen.

- Your child becomes worse.

Remember!
Contact your doctor if your child develops any of the **Call Your Doctor** symptoms.

CHAPTER 46

Puncture Wound

Definition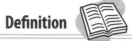

- The skin is punctured by a pointed, narrow object.

See Other Chapter If

- Animal caused it. See Chapter 52, Animal or Human Bite.
- Looks infected. See Chapter 48, Wound Infection.
- Skin is cut or scraped (not punctured). See Chapter 45, Cuts, Scrapes, and Bruises (Skin Injury).
- Foreign body (such as a sliver) remains in the skin. See Chapter 47, Skin Foreign Body or Object (Splinters).

Causes of Puncture Wounds

- **Metal:** Nail, sewing needle, pin, or tack.
- **Pencil:** Pencil lead is actually graphite (harmless). It is not poisonous lead. Even colored leads are not toxic.
- **Wood:** Toothpick.

Complications of Puncture Wounds

- **Retained foreign body (object).** This happens if part of the sharp object breaks off in the skin. Pain will not go away until it is removed.
- **Wound infection.** This happens in 4% of foot punctures. The main symptom is spreading redness 2 or 3 days after the injury.
- **Bone infection.** If the sharp object also hits a bone, the bone can become infected. Punctures of the ball of the foot are at greatest risk. Main symptoms are increased swelling and pain 2 weeks after the injury.

When to Call Your Doctor

Call 911 Now (Your Child May Need an Ambulance) If

▸ Deep puncture on the head, neck, chest, or stomach.

▸ You think your child has a life-threatening emergency.

Go to ER Now If

▸ Bleeding won't stop after 10 minutes of direct pressure.

▸ Puncture on the head, neck, chest, or stomach that could be deep.

▸ Tip of the object broke off in the body.

Call Your Doctor Now (Night or Day) If

▸ Puncture into a joint.

▸ Feels like something is still in the wound.

▸ Won't stand (bear weight or walk) on punctured foot.

▸ Needlestick from used shot needle.

▸ Sharp object or setting was very dirty (such as a playground or dirty water).

▸ No past tetanus shots.

▸ Dirt in the wound is not gone after 15 minutes of scrubbing.

▸ Severe pain doesn't improve 2 hours after taking pain medicine.

▸ Wound looks infected (spreading redness, red streaks).

▸ Fever occurs.

▸ You think your child has a serious injury.

▸ You think your child needs to be seen, and the problem is urgent.

Call Your Doctor Within 24 Hours If

▸ Last tetanus shot was more than 5 years ago.

▸ You think your child needs to be seen, but the problem is not urgent.

Call Your Doctor During Weekday Office Hours If

▸ You have other questions or concerns.

Parent Care at Home If

▸ Minor puncture wound.

Care Advice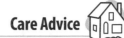

❶ What You Should Know About Puncture Wounds

- Most puncture wounds do not need to be seen.
- Here is some care advice that should help.

❷ Cleaning the Wound

- First wash off the foot, hand, or other punctured skin with soap and water.
- Then soak the puncture wound in warm, soapy water for 15 minutes.
- For any dirt or debris, gently scrub the wound surface back and forth. Use a washcloth to remove any dirt.
- If the wound rebleeds a little, that may help remove germs.

❸ Antibiotic Ointment

- Use an antibiotic ointment (such as Polysporin). No prescription is needed.
- Then, cover with a bandage (such as a Band-Aid). This helps reduce the risk of infection.
- Rewash the wound and put on antibiotic ointment every 12 hours.
- Do this for 2 days.

❹ Pain Medicine

- To help with pain, give an acetaminophen product (such as Tylenol).
- Another choice is an ibuprofen product (such as Advil).
- Use as needed.

❺ What to Expect

- Puncture wounds seal over in 1 to 2 hours.
- Pain should go away within 2 days.

❻ Call Your Doctor If

- Dirt in the wound still there after 15 minutes of scrubbing.
- Pain becomes severe.
- Looks infected (redness, red streaks, pus, or fever).
- You think your child needs to be seen.
- Your child becomes worse.

Remember!
Contact your doctor if your child develops any of the **Call Your Doctor** symptoms.

CHAPTER 47

Skin Foreign Body or Object (Splinters)

Definition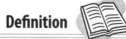

- ▶ A foreign body or object stuck in the skin.
- ▶ Some examples are a wood splinter, a fishhook, glass sliver, or a needle.

Symptoms of a Foreign Body (Object) in the Skin

- ▶ **Pain.** Most tiny slivers in the top layer of skin do not cause much pain. An example of these tiny slivers is plant stickers. Objects that are deeper or go straight down are usually painful to pressure. Objects in the foot are very painful with standing or walking.
- ▶ **Foreign body sensation.** Older children may report something being in the skin. ("I feel something in there.")

Types of Foreign Bodies (Objects)

- ▶ **Wood (organic):** Splinters, cactus spines, thorns, or toothpicks. These objects are irritating and become infected if not removed.
- ▶ **Metallic:** BBs, nails, sewing needles, pins, or tacks.
- ▶ **Fiberglass slivers.**
- ▶ **Fishhooks** may have a barbed point that makes removal difficult.
- ▶ **Glass sliver.**
- ▶ **Pencil lead** (graphite, not lead).
- ▶ **Plastic sliver.**

When to Call Your Doctor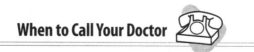

Go to ER Now If

- ▶ Object is deep (such as a needle or toothpick in the foot).

Call Your Doctor Now (Night or Day) If

▶ Object has a barb (such as a fishhook).

▶ Object is a BB.

▶ Object is causing severe pain.

▶ You want a doctor to take out the object.

▶ You tried and can't get the object out.

▶ Wound looks infected (spreading redness).

▶ Fever occurs.

▶ You think your child has a serious injury.

▶ You think your child needs to be seen, and the problem is urgent.

Call Your Doctor Within 24 Hours If

▶ Deep puncture wound and last tetanus shot was more than 5 years ago.

▶ You think your child needs to be seen, but the problem is not urgent.

Call Your Doctor During Weekday Office Hours If

▶ You have other questions or concerns.

Parent Care at Home If

▶ Tiny, pain-free slivers near the surface don't need to be removed.

▶ Tiny plant or cactus spines or fiberglass slivers need to be removed.

▶ Minor sliver, splinter, or thorn needs removal. You think you can do it at home.

Care Advice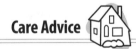

❶ Tiny, Pain-Free Slivers: Treatment

■ Tiny, pain-free slivers near the skin surface can be left in.

■ They will slowly work their way out with normal shedding of the skin.

■ Sometimes, the body will also reject them by forming a little pimple. This will drain on its own. Or you can open up the pimple. Use a clean, sterilized needle. The sliver will flow out with the pus.

❷ Tiny, Painful Plant Stickers: Treatment

■ Plant stickers or cactus spines are hard to remove. Fiberglass slivers may also be hard to get out. (**Reason:** They are fragile. Most often, they break when pressure is applied with tweezers.)

■ **Tape.** First, try touching the spot lightly with tape. Stickers should attach to the tape. You can use packaging tape, duct tape, or other sticky tape.

■ **Wax hair remover.** If tape doesn't work, use wax hair remover. Put a thin layer on. Let it air-dry for 5 minutes. You can also speed up the process with a hair dryer. Then peel it off with the stickers. Most will be removed. The others will usually work themselves out with normal shedding of the skin.

❸ Needle and Tweezers for Slivers and Splinters

■ For larger splinters, slivers, or thorns, remove with a needle and tweezers.

■ Check the tweezers first. Be certain the ends (pickups) meet exactly. If they do not, bend them. Clean the tool with rubbing alcohol before using them.

■ Briefly clean the skin around the sliver with rubbing alcohol. Do this before trying to remove it. If you don't have any, use soap and water. (**Caution:** Don't soak the spot if the foreign body is wood. **Reason:** Can cause swelling of the splinter.)

■ Use the needle to uncover the large end of the sliver. Use good lighting. A magnifying glass may help.

■ Grasp the end firmly with the tweezers. Pull it out at the same angle it went in. Get a good grip the first time. This is important for slivers that go straight into the skin. This is also important for those trapped under the fingernail.

■ For slivers under a fingernail, sometimes part of the nail must be cut away. Use fine scissors to expose the end of the sliver.

■ A sliver (when you can see all of it) can often be removed at home. Pull on the end. If the end breaks off, open the skin with a sterile needle. Go along the length of the sliver and remove it.

❹ Antibiotic Ointment

■ Wash the area with soap and water before and after removal.

■ Use an antibiotic ointment (such as Polysporin) after sliver is taken out. No prescription is needed. This will help decrease the risk of infection.

❺ Call Your Doctor If

- You can't get the object out.

- Object is out, but pain gets worse.

- Starts to look infected.

- You think your child needs to be seen.

- Your child becomes worse.

Remember!
Contact your doctor if your child develops any of the **Call Your Doctor** symptoms.

CHAPTER 48

Wound Infection

Definition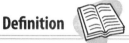

- Signs of wound infection include pus, spreading redness, increased pain or swelling, and fever.

- A break in the skin (a wound) shows signs of infection.

- Includes infected cuts, scrapes, sutured wounds, puncture wounds, and animal bites.

- Most dirty wounds become infected 24 to 72 hours later.

Symptoms of Wound Infections

- **Pus.** Pus or cloudy fluid is draining from the wound.

- **Pimple.** A pimple or yellow crust has formed on the wound.

- **Soft scab.** The scab has increased in size.

- **Red area.** Increasing redness occurs around the wound.

- **Red streak.** A red streak is spreading from the wound toward the heart.

- **More pain.** The wound has become very tender.

- **More swelling.** Pain or swelling is increasing 48 hours after the wound occurred.

- **Swollen node.** The lymph node draining that area of skin may become large and tender.

- **Fever.** A fever occurs.

- The wound hasn't healed within 10 days after the injury.

When to Call Your Doctor

Call 911 Now (Your Child May Need an Ambulance) If

- Not moving or too weak to stand.

- You think your child has a life-threatening emergency.

Call Your Doctor Now (Night or Day) If

▶ Fever occurs.

▶ Red streak runs from the wound.

▶ Spreading redness around the wound.

▶ Severe pain in the wound.

▶ Any face wound with signs of infection.

▶ No past tetanus shots.

▶ Your child looks or acts very sick.

▶ You think your child needs to be seen, and the problem is urgent.

Call Your Doctor Within 24 Hours If

▶ Pus or cloudy discharge from the wound.

▶ Wound gets more painful or tender after 2 days (48 hours).

▶ No tetanus shot in more than 5 years.

▶ You think your child needs to be seen, but the problem is not urgent.

Call Your Doctor During Weekday Office Hours If

▶ Pimple where a stitch comes through the skin.

▶ You have other questions or concerns.

Parent Care at Home If

▶ Mild redness of wound.

Care Advice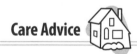

❶ What You Should Know About Normal Healing

■ Some pink or red skin on the edge of the wound is normal.

■ It's more common if the wound is sutured.

■ It's also normal for it to be swollen for a few days.

■ Your child's wound is not infected unless the redness spreads or pain increases.

■ Most dirty wounds become infected 24 to 72 hours later.

■ Here is some care advice that should help.

❷ Warm Soaks or Warm, Wet Cloth

- For any redness or other signs of early infection, use heat.

- **Open cuts or scrapes.** Soak the cut or scrape in warm water. You can also put a warm, wet cloth on the wound. Do this for 10 minutes 3 times per day. Use a warm, saltwater solution. You can make your own. Put 2 teaspoons (10 mL) of table salt in a quart (liter) of warm water.

- **Closed or sutured cuts.** Put a heating pad on the wound. You can also use a warm, moist washcloth. Do this for 10 minutes 3 times per day.

- **Cautions for sutured wounds.** Do not put anything wet on the wound for the first 24 hours. After 24 hours, your child can take brief showers. Never soak the wound before all sutures are removed.

❸ Antibiotic Ointment

- Use an antibiotic ointment (such as Polysporin).

- No prescription is needed.

- Put it on the wound 3 times a day.

- If the area could become dirty, cover it with a bandage (such as a Band-Aid).

❹ Pain Medicine

- To help with pain, give an acetaminophen product (such as Tylenol).

- Another choice is an ibuprofen product (such as Advil).

- Use as needed.

❺ Fever Medicine

- For fevers above 102°F (39°C), give an acetaminophen product (such as Tylenol).

- Another choice is an ibuprofen product (such as Advil).

- **Note:** Fevers below 102°F (39°C) are important for fighting infections.

- **For all fevers:** Keep your child well hydrated. Give lots of cold fluids.

❻ What to Expect

- Pain and swelling normally peak on day 2.

- Any redness should go away by day 4.

- Complete healing should occur by day 10.

❼ Return to School

- For true wound infections, your child can return after the fever is gone. Your child should also be taking an antibiotic by mouth for 24 hours.

- For minor redness around the wound, your child does not need to stay home.

❽ Call Your Doctor If

- Wound becomes more painful.

- Redness starts to spread.

- Pus or fever occurs.

- You think your child needs to be seen.

- Your child becomes worse.

Remember!

Contact your doctor if your child develops any of the **Call Your Doctor** symptoms.

PART 12

Skin: Widespread Symptoms

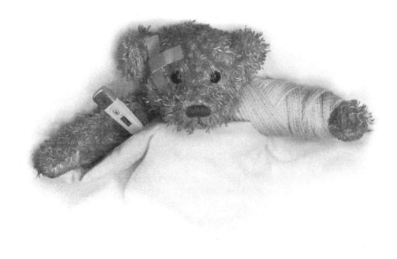

CHAPTER 49

Rash or Redness: Widespread and Cause Unknown

Definition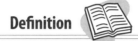

▸ Red or pink rash over large parts or most of the body (widespread).

▸ Sometimes rash just on hands, feet, and buttocks but same on both sides of the body.

▸ Small spots, large spots, or solid red skin.

See Other Chapter If

▸ Hives, especially if bumpy and itchy (Chapter 50).

▸ Sunburn (Chapter 51).

▸ Measles vaccine rash (fine, pink rash that begins 7–10 days after measles vaccine). See Chapter 57, Immunization Reactions.

Causes of Widespread Rash or Redness

▸ **Viral rash.** Most rashes are part of a viral illness. Viral rashes usually have small, pink spots. They occur on both sides of the chest, stomach, and back. Your child may also have a fever with some diarrhea or cold symptoms. Viral rashes last 2 or 3 days. More common in the summer.

▸ **Roseola.** This is the most common viral rash in the first 3 years of life.

▸ **Chickenpox.** A viral rash with a distinctive pattern. It starts as small red bumps. The bumps change to small blisters or pimples. The blisters change to open sores, and finally they scab over. The chickenpox vaccine has made the disease uncommon.

▸ **Hand-foot-and-mouth disease.** Most children have small red spots and blisters on the palms and soles. Also, the most common cause of multiple small ulcers in the mouth. The ulcers are mainly on the tongue and sides of the mouth. This is due to the Coxsackie virus. It is common between ages 1 and 5 years.

▸ **Scarlet fever.** Scarlet fever is a speckled, red rash all over. Has a sandpaper feel. Caused by strep bacteria. Starts on upper chest and quickly spreads to lower chest and stomach. No more serious than a strep throat infection without a rash.

▸ **Drug rash.** Most rashes that start while taking an antibiotic are viral rashes. Only 10% turn out to be allergic drug rashes.

▸ **Hives.** Raised, pink bumps with pale centers. Hives look like mosquito bites. Rashes that are bumpy and itchy are often hives. Most cases of hives are caused by a virus. Hives can also be an allergic reaction. (See Chapter 50, Hives, for more information.)

▸ **Heat rash.** A fine, pink rash caused by overheating. Mainly involves neck, chest, and upper back.

▸ **Insect bites.** Insect bites cause small, red bumps. Flying insects can cause many bumps on exposed skin. Nonflying insects are more likely to cause localized bumps.

▸ **Hot tub rash.** Causes small, red bumps that are painful and itchy. Mainly occurs on skin covered by a bathing suit. Rash starts 12 to 48 hours after being in a hot tub. Caused by overgrowth of bacteria in hot tubs.

▸ **Petechiae rash (serious).** Petechiae are purple- or dark red–colored tiny dots. They come from bleeding into the skin. Scattered petechiae with a fever are caused by meningococcemia until proven otherwise. This is a life-threatening bacterial infection of the bloodstream. Peak age is 3 to 6 months. Unlike most pink rashes, petechiae don't fade when pressed on.

▸ **Purpura rash (serious).** Purpura means bleeding into the skin. It looks like purple or dark red larger spots. Widespread purpura is always an emergency. It can be caused by a bacterial bloodstream infection. Rocky Mountain spotted fever is an example.

▸ **Blister rash (serious).** Widespread blisters on the skin are a serious sign. They can be caused by infections or drugs. Stevens-Johnson syndrome is an example.

▸ **Caution:** All widespread rashes with fever need to be seen. They need to be diagnosed. (**Reason:** Some serious infections can cause this type of rash.)

Drugs and Rashes

▸ Prescription medicines sometimes cause widespread rashes. Some are allergic; most are not.

▸ Nonprescription (over-the-counter) medicines rarely cause any rashes.

▸ Most rashes that occur while taking an over-the-counter medicine are viral rashes.

- Fever medicines (acetaminophen and ibuprofen) cause the most needless worry. (**Reason:** Most viral rashes start with a fever.) Hence, the child is taking a fever medicine when the rash starts.

- Drug rashes can't be diagnosed over the phone. You will need to call your doctor for advice.

Roseola: A Classic Rash

- Most children get roseola between 6 months and 3 years of age.

- **Rash:** Pink, small, flat spots on the chest and stomach. Then they spread to the face.

- **Classic feature:** 3 to 5 days of high fever without a rash or other symptoms.

- The rash starts 12 to 24 hours after the fever goes away.

- The rash lasts 1 to 3 days.

- By the time the rash appears, the child feels fine.

- **Treatment:** The rash is harmless. Creams or medicines are not needed.

Localized Versus Widespread Rash: How to Decide

- *Localized* means the rash occurs on one small part of the body. Usually, the rash is on just one side of the body. An example is a rash on one foot. (**Exceptions:** Athlete's foot can occur on both feet. Insect bites can be scattered.)

- *Widespread* means the rash occurs on larger areas. Examples are both legs or the entire back. Widespread can also mean on most of the body's surface. Widespread rashes always occur on matching (both) sides of the body. Many viral rashes are on the chest, stomach, and back.

- The cause of a widespread rash usually travels through the bloodstream. Examples are viruses, bacteria, toxins, and food or drug allergies.

- The cause of a localized rash is usually just from contact with the skin. Examples are chemicals, allergens, insect bites, ringworm fungus, bacteria, and irritants.

- This is why it's important to make this distinction.

When to Call Your Doctor

Call 911 Now (Your Child May Need an Ambulance) If

▸ Purple- or blood-colored spots or tiny dots with fever within the last 24 hours.

▸ Trouble breathing or swallowing.

▸ Not moving or too weak to stand.

▸ You think your child has a life-threatening emergency.

Go to ER Now

▸ Purple- or blood-colored spots or tiny dots without fever.

▸ Not alert when awake (out of it).

Call Your Doctor Now (Night or Day) If

▸ Bright red skin that peels off in sheets.

▸ Large blisters on the skin.

▸ Bloody crusts on the lips.

▸ Took a prescription medication within the last 3 days.

▸ Fever.

▸ Your daughter has her period and is using tampons.

▸ Your child looks or acts very sick.

▸ You think your child needs to be seen, and the problem is urgent.

Call Your Doctor Within 24 Hours If

▸ Widespread rash but none of the symptoms above. (**Reason:** All widespread rashes need to be checked by a doctor.)

Care Advice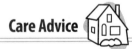

❶ What You Should Know About Widespread Rashes

■ Most rashes with small, pink spots all over are part of a viral illness.

■ This is more likely if your child has a fever. Other symptoms (like diarrhea) also point to a viral rash.

■ Here is some care advice that should help until you talk with your doctor.

❷ Non-itchy Rash Treatment

- If you suspect a heat rash, give a cool bath.

- Otherwise, no treatment is needed.

❸ Itchy Rash Treatment

- Wash the skin once with soap to remove any irritants.

- **Steroid cream.** To relieve itching, use 1% hydrocortisone cream (such as Cortaid). Put it on the itchiest areas. No prescription is needed. Do this 3 times per day.

- **Cool bath.** For flare-ups of itching, give your child a cool bath. Do not use soap. Do this for 10 minutes. (**Caution:** Avoid any chill.) (**Option:** Can add 2 ounces [60 mL] of baking soda per tub.)

- **Scratching.** Try to keep your child from scratching. Cut the fingernails short. (**Reason:** Prevents a skin infection from bacteria.)

- **Allergy medicine.** If itching persists, use an allergy medicine until you see your doctor. Benadryl can be used for a few days. **Age limit:** 1 year and older. A long-acting allergy medicine, such as Zyrtec, is preferred. **Age limit:** 2 years and older.

❹ Fever Medicine

- For fevers above 102°F (39°C), give an acetaminophen product (such as Tylenol).

- Another choice is an ibuprofen product (such as Advil).

- **Note:** Fevers below 102°F (39°C) are important for fighting infections.

- **For all fevers:** Keep your child well hydrated. Give lots of cold fluids.

❺ Return to School

- Most viral rashes can be spread to others (especially if a fever is present).

- If your child has a fever, avoid contact with other children. Avoid pregnant women until a diagnosis is made.

- For minor rashes, your child can return to school after the fever is gone.

- For major rashes, your child can return to school after the rash is gone. If your doctor has given medical clearance, your child can return sooner.

❻ What to Expect

- Most viral rashes go away within 48 hours.

❼ Call Your Doctor If

■ You think your child needs to be seen.

■ Your child becomes worse.

Remember!
Contact your doctor if your child develops any of the **Call Your Doctor** symptoms.

CHAPTER 50

Hives

Definition

- A rash made up of raised, pink bumps.
- Most often, rash is very itchy.

See Other Chapter If

- Does not look like hives. See Chapter 49, Rash or Redness: Widespread and Cause Unknown.
- Mosquito bites are the cause. See Chapter 54, Mosquito Bite.

Symptoms of Hives

- Raised, pink bumps with pale centers (welts).
- Hives look like mosquito bites.
- Sizes of hives vary from ½ in (1.3 cm) to several inches (centimeters) across.
- Shapes and location of hives can be different. They can also change frequently.
- Itchy rash.

Causes of Widespread Hives

- **Viral infection.** The most common cause of hives all over the body is a viral infection. Research has confirmed this. Other symptoms such as a fever, cough, or diarrhea are also present. The hives may last 3 days. This is not an allergy.
- **Bacterial infection.** Some bacterial infections can also cause hives. A common example is strep infection. Hives are also seen with bladder infections.
- **Drug reaction.** An example is a penicillin rash. Most rashes that start while taking an antibiotic are viral rashes. Allergy test results are normal 90% of the time. Only 10% of the time they turn out to be a drug allergy.
- **Food reaction.** May be an allergy or a coincidence. If the food is a high-risk one (such as peanuts), consult an allergist. Hives from foods usually resolve in 6 hours. Hives from infections last for days. Only 3% of hives are due to a food.

- **Bee sting.** Widespread hives after a sting may be part of a serious allergic reaction. Need to consult an allergist.

- **Anaphylactic reaction (very serious).** Sudden onset of hives with trouble breathing or swallowing. This is a severe allergic reaction to an allergic food or drug. Most often begins within 30 minutes of swallowing the substance. Always within 2 hours of exposure.

- **Unknown.** More than 30% of the time, the cause of hives is not found.

Causes of Localized Hives

- **Irritants.** Hives in just one spot are usually due to skin contact with an irritant. This is not an allergy.

- **Plants.** Many plants cause skin reactions. Sap from evergreens can cause local hives.

- **Pollen.** Playing in the grass can cause hives on exposed skin.

- **Pet saliva.** Some people get hives where a dog or cat has licked them.

- **Food.** Some children get hives if a food is rubbed on the skin. An example could be a fresh fruit. Some babies get hives around their mouth from drooling a new food.

- **Insect bite.** Local hives are a reaction to the insect's saliva. Can be very large without being an allergy.

- **Bee sting.** This is a reaction to the bee's venom. Can be very large without being an allergy.

- **Note:** Localized hives are not caused by drugs, infections, or swallowed foods. These get into the bloodstream and cause widespread hives.

First Aid for Anaphylaxis: Epinephrine

- Anaphylaxis is a life-threatening allergic reaction.

- If you have epinephrine (such as EpiPen or Auvi-Q), give it now.

- Do this while calling 911.

- More than 66 lb (30 kg): Give 0.3 mg EpiPen.

- Between 22 and 66 lb (10–30 kg): Give 0.15 mg EpiPen Jr.

- Less than 22 pounds (10 kg): Give dose advised by your doctor.

- Give the shot into the upper, outer thigh in the leg straight down.

- Can be given through clothing if needed.

- A second shot should be given if no improvement in 10 minutes.

- Benadryl: After giving the EpiPen, give Benadryl by mouth. Do this if your child is able to swallow.

When to Call Your Doctor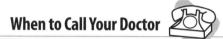

Call 911 Now (Your Child Nay Need an Ambulance) If

- Hives and life-threatening allergic reaction to similar substance in the past and exposure less than 2 hours ago.

- Trouble breathing or wheezing.

- Hoarse voice or cough start suddenly.

- Trouble swallowing, drooling, or slurred speech starts suddenly.

- You think your child has a life-threatening emergency.

Go to ER Now If

- Hives start within 2 hours after a bee sting.

Call Your Doctor Now (Night or Day) If

- Hives start after eating a high-risk food. High-risk foods include nuts, fish, shell-fish, or eggs.

- Hives started after taking a prescription medicine.

- **Age:** Younger than 1 year with hives all over.

- Your child looks or acts very sick.

- You think your child needs to be seen, and the problem is urgent.

Call Your Doctor Within 24 Hours If

- Hives started after taking an over-the-counter medicine.

- Severe hives (such as eyes swollen shut or very itchy).

- Fever or joint swelling is present.

- Stomach pain or vomiting is present.

- You think your child needs to be seen, but the problem is not urgent.

Call Your Doctor During Weekday Office Hours If

▶ Hives make it hard to go to school or do other normal activities. (**Note:** Taking Benadryl for 24 hours has not helped.)

▶ Food could be the cause.

▶ Had hives 3 or more times and the cause is not clear.

▶ Hives last more than 1 week.

▶ You have other questions or concerns.

Parent Care at Home If

▶ Hives with no complications.

Care Advice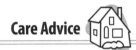

❶ Hives on Only One Part of the Body: What You Should Know

■ Most are caused by skin contact with an irritant. Examples are plants, pollen, and food or pet saliva.

■ Localized hives are not caused by drugs, infections, or swallowed foods. They are also not an allergy.

■ Wash the allergic substance off the skin with soap and water.

■ If itchy, use a cold pack for 20 minutes. You can also rub the hives with an ice cube for 10 minutes.

■ Hives on just one part of the body should go away on their own. They don't need Benadryl.

■ They should go away in a few hours.

❷ Hives All Over the Body: What You Should Know

■ More than 10% of children get hives one or more times.

■ Most widespread hives are caused by a viral infection. This is not due to an allergy. Less than 10% are an allergic reaction to a food, a drug, or an insect bite. Often, the cause is not found.

■ Here is some care advice that should help.

❸ Allergy Medicine for Hives All Over the Body

- Give Benadryl 4 times per day for hives all over that itch. No prescription is needed. **Age limit:** 1 year or older.

- Use the allergy medicine until the hives are gone for 12 hours.

- If the hives last more than a few days, switch to a long-acting antihistamine, such as Zyrtec. No prescription is needed. **Age limit:** 2 years and older.

- **Caution:** Call your doctor for advice if younger than 1 year.

❹ Hives Caused by Foods

- Foods can cause widespread hives.

- Sometimes, the hives are around just the mouth.

- Hives from foods usually last just a short time. They are often gone in less than 6 hours.

❺ Cool Bath for Itching

- To help with itching, give a cool bath. Do this for 10 minutes. (**Caution:** Avoid causing a chill.)

- Can also rub very itchy spots with an ice cube for 10 minutes.

❻ Wash Allergens Off the Body

- Give a bath or shower if caused by pollens or animal contact.

- Change clothes.

❼ Stay Away From Allergens

- If you know what is causing the hives, avoid this substance. An example is certain foods.

- Help your child stay away from this allergen in the future.

❽ Return to School

- Hives cannot be spread to others.

- Your child can go back to school once feeling better. The hives shouldn't keep your child from doing normal activities.

- For hives from an infection, can go back after the fever is gone. Your child should feel well enough to join in normal activities.

❾ What to Expect

- Hives all over from a viral illness normally come and go.
- They may last for 3 or 4 days. Then, they go away.
- Most children get hives once.

❿ Call Your Doctor If

- Severe hives don't improve after 2 doses of Benadryl.
- Itch not better after 24 hours on Benadryl.
- Hives last more than 1 week.
- You think your child needs to be seen.
- Your child becomes worse.

Remember!
Contact your doctor if your child develops any of the **Call Your Doctor** symptoms.

CHAPTER 51

Sunburn

Definition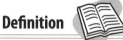

- ▸ Red or blistered skin from too much sun.
- ▸ Redness, pain, and swelling starts at 4 hours after being in the sun.
- ▸ It peaks at 24 hours and starts to get better after 48 hours.

See Other Chapter If

- ▸ Sunburn-like rash but no sun exposure. See Chapter 49, Rash or Redness: Widespread and Cause Unknown.

Severity of Sunburn

- ▸ Most sunburns are a first-degree burn that turns the skin pink or red.
- ▸ Prolonged sun exposure can cause blistering and a second-degree burn.
- ▸ Sunburn never causes a third-degree burn or scarring.

Causes of Sunburn

- ▸ **Direct sun exposure.** (**Caution:** Clouds don't help. Seventy percent of UV [ultraviolet] light still gets through on cloudy days.)
- ▸ **Reflected sun rays.** From snow, 80% is reflected; from sand, 20%; from water, only 5%.
- ▸ **Tanning or sun lamp.**
- ▸ **Tanning bed.** A common cause in teens.

Ibuprofen to Reduce Pain and Other Symptoms

- ▸ Sunburn is an inflammatory reaction of the skin.
- ▸ Ibuprofen is a drug that can block this reaction. It can reduce redness and swelling. But, it needs to be started early.
- ▸ Redness (sunburn) is often not seen until 4 hours after being in the sun. Pain and redness keep getting worse. They don't peak for 24 to 36 hours. Many

parents are surprised when their child gets a sunburn. (**Reason:** There are no warning signs while the burn is occurring.)

▸ **Lesson:** If you think your child got too much sun, start ibuprofen then. Give it 3 times per day for 2 days. Don't wait for redness.

When to Call Your Doctor

Call 911 Now (Your Child May Need an Ambulance) If

▸ Passed out or too weak to stand.

▸ You think your child has a life-threatening emergency.

Call Your Doctor Now (Night or Day) If

▸ Fever above 104°F (40°C).

▸ Can't look at lights because of eye pain.

▸ Fever and sunburn looks infected (spreading redness more than 48 hours after the sunburn).

▸ Your child looks or acts very sick.

▸ You think your child needs to be seen, and the problem is urgent.

Call Your Doctor Within 24 Hours If

▸ Sunburn pain is severe and not better after using this chapter's Care Advice.

▸ Large blisters (more than ½ in or 1.3 cm).

▸ Many small blisters.

▸ Blisters on the face.

▸ Swollen feet make it hard to walk.

▸ Looks infected (draining pus, red streaks, and pain worse after day 2) and no fever.

▸ You think your child needs to be seen, but the problem is not urgent.

Call Your Doctor During Weekday Office Hours If

▸ Itchy rashes in sun-exposed skin occur many times.

▸ You have other questions or concerns.

Parent Care at Home If

▸ Mild sunburn.

Care Advice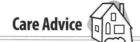

Treating Mild Sunburn

❶ What You Should Know About Sunburns

- Most sunburns do not blister.

- Most blisters can be treated without needing to see a doctor.

- Here is some care advice that should help.

❷ Ibuprofen for Pain

- For pain relief, give an ibuprofen product (such as Advil). Start this as soon as you can.

- Give every 6 to 8 hours.

- **Reason:** If started within 6 hours, it can greatly limit the pain and swelling. Must give for 2 days.

- **Caution:** Not approved for babies younger than 6 months.

❸ Steroid Cream for Pain

- Use 1% hydrocortisone cream (such as Cortaid) as soon as possible. No prescription is needed.

- Put it on 3 times per day.

- If used early and continued for 2 days, it may reduce swelling and pain.

- Use a moisturizing or an aloe vera cream until you can get some steroid cream.

- Use only creams. Avoid putting ointments on red skin. (**Reason:** They can block sweat glands.)

- Burned skin can be very painful. Covering it with a cream can give great relief.

❹ Cool Baths for Pain

- Apply cool, wet washcloths to the burned area. Do this several times a day to reduce pain and burning.

- For larger sunburns, give cool baths for 10 minutes. (**Caution:** Avoid any chill.) Can add 2 ounces (60 mL) baking soda per tub.

- Do not use soap on the sunburn.

❺ Fluids: Offer More

- Offer extra water, especially on the first day.

- This helps replace fluids lost because of the sunburn.

- This will also help prevent dehydration and dizziness.

❻ Blisters: Don't Open

- **Caution:** Leave closed blisters alone. (**Reason:** To prevent infection.)

- For broken blisters, trim off the dead skin. Use fine scissors cleaned with rubbing alcohol.

❼ Antibiotic Ointment for Open Blisters

- For any large, open blisters, use an antibiotic ointment (such as Polysporin). No prescription is needed.

- Remove it with warm water. Then, reapply it 2 times a day for 3 days.

❽ What to Expect

- Pain stops after 2 or 3 days.

- Peeling occurs day 5, 6, or 7.

❾ Call Your Doctor If

- Pain becomes severe.

- Sunburn looks infected.

- You think your child needs to be seen.

- Your child becomes worse.

Preventing Sunburn

❶ Sunscreens

- Use a sunscreen with an SPF (sun protection factor) of 15 or higher. Fair-skinned children need a sunscreen with an SPF of 30. This is especially true if your child has red or blond hair.

- Put sunscreen on 30 minutes before exposure to the sun. This gives it time to get down into the skin. Give special attention to areas most likely to become sunburned. Examples are the nose, ears, cheeks, and shoulders.

- Reapply sunscreen every 3 to 4 hours. Apply often while swimming or if your child is sweating a lot. A "waterproof" sunscreen stays on for about 30 minutes in water.

- Most people use too little sunscreen. The average adult requires 1 ounce (30 mL) of sunscreen at a time.

- The best way to prevent skin cancer is to prevent sunburns.

❷ Babies and Sunscreens

- The skin of babies is thinner than the skin of older children. It is more sensitive to the sun. Sunburns can occur quickly.

- Sun avoidance is best for babies younger than 6 months. Stay in the shade.

- Sun avoidance or sunproof clothing is best for infants and children 6 months to 3 years. If they have to be in the sun, use clothes that fully cover the arms and legs. Also, have your child wear a hat with a brim. Apply sunscreen to exposed skin. Use a stroller with a canopy.

- When a sunscreen is needed, infants can use adult sunscreens. The US Food and Drug Administration hasn't approved their use in babies younger than 6 months. However, the American Academy of Pediatrics supports their use at this age. There are no reported harmful side effects from today's sunscreens.

❸ Protect Lips, Nose, and Eyes

- To prevent sunburned lips, apply a lip coating that contains sunscreen.

- If the nose or some other area has been burned often, protect it completely. Use zinc or titanium oxide ointment.

- Protect your child's eyes from the sun's rays and cataracts with good sunglasses.

❹ High-Risk Children

- Some children are at higher risk for sunburn. If your child has red or blond hair, she is at higher risk. Fair-skinned children and children who never tan are also at higher risk.

- These children need to use a sunscreen even for brief exposures.

- They should avoid sun exposure whenever possible.

❺ High-Risk Time of Day

- Avoid exposure to the sun during the hours of 11:00 am to 3:00 pm. This is when the sun's rays are most intense.

- **Caution:** When the sky is overcast, more than 70% of the sun's rays still get through the clouds.

Remember!
Contact your doctor if your child develops any of the **Call Your Doctor** symptoms.

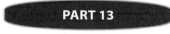

Bites or Stings

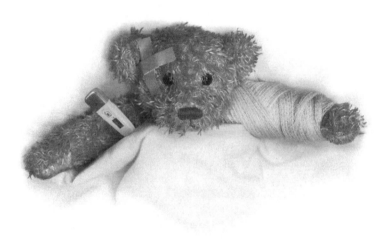

CHAPTER 52

Animal or Human Bite

Definition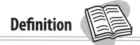

▸ Bite from a pet, wild animal, or a human.

▸ Any animal-related skin injury.

Types of Wounds

▸ **Bruise.** No break is in the skin. No risk of infection.

▸ **Scrape (abrasion) or scratch.** A wound that doesn't go all the way through the skin. Low chance of infection. Antibiotic drugs are not needed.

▸ **Cut (laceration).** A wound that goes through the skin to the fat or muscle tissue. Some chance of infection. Most need to be seen. Cleaning the wound can help prevent this. Antibiotic drugs may be needed.

▸ **Puncture wound.** These wounds break through the skin. Greater risk of infection. Puncture wounds from cat bites are more likely to get infected. Antibiotic drugs may be needed.

▸ **Wound infection.** This is the main risk of an animal bite. The main finding is redness around the bite and pain. It starts 1 to 3 days after the bite. It can often be prevented by early, careful cleaning of the bite. This is why most animal bites need to be seen.

Types of Animal Bites

▸ **Rabies-prone wild animal bites.** Rabies is a disease that can kill people. Bites or scratches from any large wild animal can pass on rabies. Animals at highest risk for rabies are bats, skunks, raccoons, foxes, or coyotes. These animals may spread rabies even if they have no symptoms.

▸ **Small wild animal bites.** Small animals such as mice, rats, moles, or gophers do not carry rabies. Chipmunks, prairie dogs, and rabbits also do not carry rabies. **Exception:** One of these small animals actually attacks a human (an unprovoked bite). Sometimes, their bites can get infected. Squirrels rarely carry rabies but have not transmitted it to humans.

- **Large pet animal bites.** Most bites from pets are from dogs or cats. Bites from other animals such as horses can be handled by using this chapter. Dogs and cats are free of rabies in most cities in the United States and Canada. Stray animals are always at risk for rabies until proven otherwise. Cats and dogs that always stay indoors should be safe. The main risk in pet bites is wound infection, not rabies. Cat bites become infected more often than dog bites. Cat scratches can get infected just like a bite because their claws can be dirty with saliva.

- **Small indoor pet animal bites.** Small indoor pets are not at risk for rabies. Examples of these pets are gerbils, hamsters, guinea pigs, or mice. Tiny puncture wounds from these small animals also don't need to be seen. They carry a small risk for wound infections.

- **Human bites.** Most human bites occur during fights, especially in teens. Sometimes a fist is cut when it strikes a tooth. Human bites are more likely to become infected than animal bites. Bites on the hands are at higher risk. Many toddler bites are safe because they don't break the skin.

- **Bats and rabies.** In the United States, 90% of cases of rabies in humans are caused by bats. Bats have spread rabies without a visible bite mark.

Animals at Risk for Rabies

- Bat, skunk, raccoon, fox, or coyote.
- Other large wild animals.
- Pets that have never had rabies shots and spend time outdoors.
- In the United States, rabies occurs 4 times more in cats than dogs.
- Outdoor animals who are sick or stray.
- Dogs or cats in countries that do not require rabies shots.
- In the United States and Canada, bites from most city dogs and cats are safe (free of rabies).
- In the United States, there are 2 to 3 deaths from rabies per year in humans.

First Aid for All Bites and Scratches

- Wash all bite wounds and scratches right now with soap and warm water. (**Reason:** To prevent wound infections.)

First Aid for Bleeding

- Place a gauze pad or clean cloth on top of the wound.
- Press down firmly on the place that is bleeding.

▸ This is called *direct pressure*. It is the best way to stop bleeding.

▸ Keep using pressure until the bleeding stops.

▸ If bleeding does not stop, press on a slightly different spot.

When to Call Your Doctor

Call 911 Now (Your Child May Need an Ambulance) If

▸ Major bleeding that can't be stopped.

▸ Not moving or too weak to stand.

▸ You think your child has a life-threatening emergency.

Go to ER Now If

▸ Bleeding won't stop after 10 minutes of direct pressure.

▸ Any scratch or cut from an animal at risk for rabies.

Call Your Doctor Now (Night or Day) If

▸ Wild animal bite that breaks the skin.

▸ Pet animal (such as dog or cat) bite that breaks the skin. (**Exception:** Minor scratches that don't go through the skin.)

▸ Puncture wound (holes through the skin) from a cat's teeth or claws.

▸ Puncture wound (holes through the skin) of a hand or the face.

▸ Human bite that breaks the skin.

▸ Finger or hand swelling that follows an animal bite.

▸ Bite looks infected (redness or red streaks) or your child has a fever.

▸ Bat contact or exposure, even without a bite mark.

▸ Contact with a rabies-prone animal, even without a bite mark.

▸ Minor cut or scrape and no past tetanus shots.

▸ Your child looks or acts very sick.

▸ You think your child needs to be seen, and the problem is urgent.

Call Your Doctor Within 24 Hours If

▸ Last tetanus shot was more than 5 years ago.

▸ You think your child needs to be seen, but the problem is not urgent.

Call Your Doctor During Weekday Office Hours If

▶ You have other questions or concerns.

Parent Care at Home If

▶ Bite did not break the skin or is only a bruise.

▶ Minor scratches that don't go through the skin from a pet.

▶ Tiny puncture wound from small pet, such as a hamster or puppy. (**Exception:** Cat puncture wound.)

Care Advice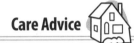

❶ What You Should Know About Bites

■ Bites that don't break the skin can't become infected.

■ Cuts and punctures are always at risk for infection.

■ Here is some care advice that should help.

❷ Clean the Bite

■ Wash all wounds right now with soap and water for 5 minutes.

■ Also, flush well under running water for a few minutes. (**Reason:** Can prevent many wound infections.)

❸ Bleeding: How to Stop It

■ For any bleeding, put pressure on the wound.

■ Use a gauze pad or clean cloth.

■ Press for 10 minutes or until the bleeding has stopped.

❹ Antibiotic Ointment

■ For small cuts, use an antibiotic ointment (such as Polysporin). No prescription is needed.

■ Put it on the cut 3 times a day.

■ Do this for 3 days.

❺ Pain Medicine

■ To help with pain, give an acetaminophen product (such as Tylenol).

■ Another choice is an ibuprofen product (such as Advil).

■ Use as needed.

❻ Cold Pack for Pain

- For pain or bruising, use a cold pack. You can also use ice wrapped in a wet cloth. Apply it to the bruise once for 20 minutes. (**Reason:** Helps with bleeding, pain, and swelling.)

❼ What to Expect

- Most scratches, scrapes, and other minor bites heal fine in 5 to 7 days.

❽ Call Your Doctor If

- Bite starts to look infected (pus, redness, and red streaks).

- Fever occurs.

- You think your child needs to be seen.

- Your child becomes worse.

Remember!
Contact your doctor if your child develops any of the **Call Your Doctor** symptoms.

CHAPTER 53

Bee or Yellow Jacket Sting

Definition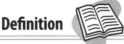

- ▸ Sting from a bee, hornet, wasp, or yellow jacket.
- ▸ Main symptoms: pain and redness.

Cause of Bee Sting Reactions

- ▸ Bee stinger injects venom into the skin.
- ▸ Venom is what causes symptoms.

Local Skin Reactions to the Sting

- ▸ Main symptoms are pain, itching, swelling, and redness at the sting site.
- ▸ **Pain.** Severe pain or burning at the site lasts 1 to 2 hours. Itching often follows the pain.
- ▸ **Swelling.** Bee sting may swell for 48 hours after the sting. Swelling can be small or large. Stings on the face can cause a lot of swelling around the eye. It looks bad but is not serious. Swelling may last for 7 days.
- ▸ **Redness.** Bee stings are often red. That doesn't mean they are infected. Infections rarely happen with stings. The redness can last 3 days.

Anaphylactic Reaction to the Sting

- ▸ A severe life-threatening allergic reaction is called *anaphylaxis.*
- ▸ The main symptom is hives with trouble breathing and swallowing. It starts within 2 hours of the sting.
- ▸ This severe reaction to bee stings occurs in 4 out of 1,000 children.
- ▸ **Hives.** After a bee sting, some children develop hives all over or face swelling. Hives or face swelling alone may be able to be treated at home. But, at times, these symptoms can also lead to anaphylaxis. Be sure to call your doctor now to help decide whether anaphylaxis is possible.

Prevention of Bee Stings

▶ Don't go barefoot if bees are around.

▶ Be careful in gardens and orchards.

▶ Insect repellents do not work against these stinging insects.

First Aid for Anaphylaxis: Epinephrine

▶ Anaphylaxis is a life-threatening allergic reaction.

▶ If you have epinephrine (such as EpiPen or Auvi-Q), give it now.

▶ Do this while calling 911.

▶ More than 66 lb (30 kg): Give 0.3 mg EpiPen.

▶ Between 22 and 66 lb (10–30 kg): Give 0.15 mg EpiPen Jr.

▶ Less than 22 lb (10 kg): Give dose advised by your doctor.

▶ Give shot into the upper, outer thigh in the leg straight down.

▶ Can be given through clothing if needed.

▶ A second shot should be given if no improvement in 10 minutes.

▶ Benadryl: After giving the EpiPen, give Benadryl by mouth. Do this if your child is able to swallow.

When to Call Your Doctor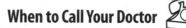

Call 911 Now (Your Child May Need an Ambulance) If

▶ Past severe allergic reaction to bee stings (not just hives) and stung less than 2 hours ago.

▶ Wheezing or trouble breathing.

▶ Hoarseness, cough, or tightness in the throat or chest.

▶ Trouble swallowing or drooling.

▶ Speech is slurred.

▶ Acts or talks confused.

▶ Passed out or too weak to stand.

▶ You think your child has a life-threatening emergency.

Go to ER Now If

▶ Hives or swelling all over the body.

Call Your Doctor Now (Night or Day) If

▶ Sting inside the mouth.

▶ Sting on the eye.

▶ Stomach pain or vomiting.

▶ More than 5 stings for each 10 lb (5 kg) of weight (in teens, more than 50 stings).

▶ Fever and sting looks infected (spreading redness).

▶ Your child looks or acts very sick.

▶ You think your child needs to be seen, and the problem is urgent.

Call Your Doctor Within 24 Hours If

▶ More than 48 hours since the sting and redness getting larger. (**Note:** Infection is not common. It does not start until at least 24 – 48 hours after the sting. Redness that starts in the first 24 hours is due to venom.)

▶ Swelling is huge (4 in or 10.2 cm). It spreads across a joint such as the wrist.

▶ You think your child needs to be seen, but the problem is not urgent.

Call Your Doctor During Weekday Office Hours If

▶ You have other questions or concerns.

Parent Care at Home If

▶ Normal reaction to bee or yellow jacket sting.

Care Advice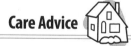

❶ What You Should Know About Bee Stings

■ Bee stings are common.

■ Main symptoms are pain and redness.

■ Swelling can be large. This does not mean it's an allergy.

■ Over 95% of stings are from honeybees or yellow jackets.

■ Here is some care advice that should help.

❷ Try to Remove the Stinger (if Present)

- Only honeybees leave a stinger.

- The stinger looks like a tiny black dot in the sting.

- Use a fingernail or credit card edge to scrape it off.

- If the stinger is below the skin surface, leave it alone. It will come out with normal skin shedding.

❸ Meat Tenderizer for Pain Relief

- Make a meat tenderizer paste with a little water. Use a cotton ball to rub it on the sting. Do this once for 20 minutes. (**Reason:** This may neutralize venom and reduce pain and swelling.) **Caution:** Do not use near the eye.

- If you don't have any, use an aluminum-based deodorant. You can also put a baking soda paste on the sting. Do this for 20 minutes.

❹ Cold Pack for Pain

- If pain does not improve after using the meat tenderizer paste, massage the spot of the sting with an ice cube.

- Do this for 10 minutes.

❺ Pain Medicine

- To help with pain, give an acetaminophen product (such as Tylenol).

- Another choice is an ibuprofen product (such as Advil).

- Use as needed.

❻ Steroid Cream for Itching

- For itching or swelling, put 1% hydrocortisone cream (such as Cortaid) on the sting.

- No prescription is needed.

- Use 3 times per day.

❼ Allergy Medicine for Itching

- For hives or severe itching, give a dose of Benadryl. **Age limit:** 1 year and older.

❽ What to Expect

- Severe pain or burning at the site lasts 1 to 2 hours.

- Normal swelling from venom can increase for 48 hours after the sting.

- Redness can last 3 days.

- Swelling can last 7 days.

❾ Call Your Doctor If

- Trouble breathing or swallowing occurs (mainly during the 2 hours after the sting). **Call 911.**

- Redness gets larger after 2 days.

- Swelling becomes huge.

- Sting starts to look infected.

- You think your child needs to be seen.

- Your child becomes worse.

> ### Remember!
> Contact your doctor if your child develops any of the **Call Your Doctor** symptoms.

CHAPTER 54

Mosquito Bite

Definition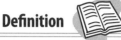

▶ Bites from a mosquito.

▶ Cause itchy, red bumps.

▶ Often they look like a hive.

▶ West Nile virus (WNV) questions.

Types of Reactions to Mosquito Bites

▶ **Red bumps.** In North America, mosquito bites are mainly an annoyance. They cause itchy red skin bumps. Often, the bite looks like hives (either one large one or several small ones).

▶ When a mosquito bites, its secretions are injected into the skin. Red bumps are the body's reaction to this process.

▶ Suspect mosquito bites if bites are on other parts of the body. Most bites occur on exposed parts, such as the face and arms.

▶ **Swelling.** Bites of the upper face can cause severe swelling around the eye. This can last for several days. With bites, the swelling can be pink as well as large (especially in children aged 1–5 years).

▶ **Disease.** Rarely, the mosquito can carry a serious blood-borne disease. In the United States and Canada, this is mainly WNV. In Africa and South America, mosquitos also carry malaria and yellow fever.

▶ **Prevention.** Insect repellents can prevent mosquito bites. Use DEET (applied to skin) and permethrin (applied to clothing).

Cause of Mosquito Bite Reaction

▶ Skin bumps are the body's reaction to the mosquito's saliva.

▶ While it's sucking blood, some of its secretions get mixed in.

Mosquito Life Cycle

- Only female mosquitoes bite. They need a blood meal to produce eggs. The female may bite 20 times before she finds a small blood vessel. She then sips blood for 90 seconds.

- Males eat flower nectar and plant juices.

- One hundred seventy species of mosquito are in North America.

- At a far distance, they are attracted by smell (breath odors, sweat, and perfumes). They can smell up to 120 ft (36 m). At a close distance, they are attracted by body heat and movement.

Risk Factors for Increased Mosquito Bites

- Warmer body temperature.

- Males more than females.

- Children more than adults.

- Breath odors.

- Sweating.

- Perfumed soaps and shampoos.

Complications of Insect Bites

- **Impetigo.** A local bacterial infection. Causes sores, soft scabs, and pus. Caused by scratching or picking at the bites. More common in itchy bites.

- **Cellulitis.** The bacterial infection spreads into the skin. Causes redness spreading out from the bite. This red area is painful to the touch.

- **Lymphangitis.** The bacterial infection spreads up the lymph channels. Causes a red line that goes up the arm or leg. More serious because the infection can get into the bloodstream. (This is called *sepsis.*)

First Aid for Anaphylaxis: Epinephrine

- Anaphylaxis is a life-threatening allergic reaction.

- If you have epinephrine (such as EpiPen or Auvi-Q), give it now.

- Do this while calling 911.

- More than 66 lb (30 kg): Give 0.3 mg EpiPen.

- Between 22 and 66 lb (10–30 kg): Give 0.15 mg EpiPen Jr.

- Less than 22 lb (10 kg): Give dose advised by your doctor.

- Give shot into the upper, outer thigh in the leg straight down.

- Can be given through clothing if needed.

- Benadryl: After giving the EpiPen, give Benadryl by mouth. Do this if your child is able to swallow.

When to Call Your Doctor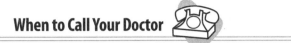

Call 911 Now (Your Child May Need an Ambulance) If

- Life-threatening allergic reaction suspected. Symptoms include sudden onset of trouble breathing or swallowing.

- Can't wake up.

- You think your child has a life-threatening emergency.

Go to ER Now If

- Hard to wake up.

- Acts or talks confused.

- Can't walk or can barely walk.

- Stiff neck (can't touch chin to chest).

Call Your Doctor Now (Night or Day) If

- Spreading red area or streak with fever.

- Your child looks or acts very sick.

- You think your child needs to be seen, and the problem is urgent.

Call Your Doctor Within 24 Hours If

- Painful, spreading redness started more than 24 hours after the bite. (**Note:** Any redness starting in the first 24 hours is a reaction to the bite.)

- More than 48 hours since the bite and red area gets larger.

- Unexplained fever and recent travel outside the country to a high-risk area.

- You think your child needs to be seen, but the problem is not urgent.

Call Your Doctor During Weekday Office Hours If

- Pregnant and recently traveled to or lives in a place with a Zika virus outbreak.

- Scab that looks infected (drains pus or gets bigger) not better with antibiotic ointment.

▸ Severe itching not better after 24 hours of steroid cream.

▸ You have other questions or concerns.

Parent Care at Home If

▸ Normal mosquito bite.

▸ Questions about WNV.

▸ Questions about insect repellents (such as DEET).

Care Advice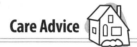

Treatment for Mosquito Bites

❶ What You Should Know

- In the United States and Canada, mosquito bites rarely carry any disease.

- They cause itchy, red skin bumps.

- Most of the time, the bumps are less than ½ in (1.3 cm) in size. In young children, they can be larger.

- Some even have a small water blister in the center.

- A large hive at the bite does not mean your child has an allergy.

- Redness does not mean the bite is infected.

- Here is some care advice that should help.

❷ Steroid Cream for Itching

- To relieve itching, use 1% hydrocortisone cream (such as Cortaid). No prescription is needed. Put it on 3 times a day until the itch is gone. If you don't have any, use a baking soda paste until you can get some.

- If neither is available, use ice in a wet washcloth for 20 minutes.

- Also, firm, sharp, direct, steady pressure on the bite for 10 seconds can help relieve the itch. A fingernail, pen cap, or other object can be used.

❸ Allergy Medicine for Itching

- If the bite is still itchy, try an allergy medicine (such as Benadryl). No prescription is needed. **Age limit:** 1 year and older.

- Sometimes it helps, especially in children with allergies.

❹ Try Not to Scratch

- Cut the fingernails short.

- Help your child not to scratch.

- **Reason:** Prevents a skin infection at the bite site.

❺ Antibiotic Ointment

- If the bite has a scab and looks infected, use an antibiotic ointment. An example is Polysporin.

- No prescription is needed. Use 3 times per day. (**Note:** Usually, infection is caused by scratching bites with dirty fingers.)

- Cover the scab with a bandage (such as a Band-Aid). This will help prevent scratching and spread.

- Wash the sore and use the antibiotic ointment 3 times per day. Do this until healed.

❻ What to Expect

- Most mosquito bites itch for 3 or 4 days.

- Any pinkness or redness usually lasts 3 or 4 days.

- Swelling may last 7 days.

- Bites of the upper face can cause severe swelling around the eye. This does not hurt the vision and is harmless.

- Swelling is often worse in the morning after lying down all night. It will improve after standing for a few hours.

❼ Call Your Doctor If

- Bite looks infected (red area gets larger after 48 hours).

- Bite becomes painful.

- You think your child needs to be seen.

- Your child becomes worse.

West Nile Virus Questions

❶ West Nile Virus: What You Should Know

- West Nile virus is a disease carried by mosquitoes. It can be spread to humans through a mosquito bite.

  - ʾout 1% of mosquitoes carry this disease.

- Of people who get WNV, less than 1% get the serious kind.
- Here are some facts that should help.

❷ Symptoms of West Nile Virus

- **No symptoms:** 80% of WNV infections.
- **Mild symptoms:** 20% of infections. Symptoms include fever, headache, and body aches. Some have a skin rash. These symptoms last 3 to 6 days. They go away without any treatment. This is called *WNV fever.*
- **Serious symptoms:** Less than 1% (1 out of 150) of WNV infections. Symptoms are high fever, stiff neck, confusion, coma, seizures, and muscle weakness. The muscle weakness is often on just one side. The cause is infection of the brain (*encephalitis*) or spinal cord (*viral meningitis*).
- **Death:** 10% of those who need to be in the hospital.
- Child cases are most often mild. Most serious cases occur in people older than 60.

❸ Diagnosis of West Nile Virus

- Children with mild symptoms do not need to see a doctor. They do not need any special tests.
- Children with severe symptoms (*encephalitis* or *viral meningitis*) need to see a doctor right away. Special tests of the blood and spinal fluid will be done to confirm the virus.
- Pregnant or breastfeeding women need to see a doctor if they have symptoms.

❹ Treatment of West Nile Virus

- No special treatment is needed after a mosquito bite.
- There is no special treatment or antiviral drug for WNV symptoms.
- People with serious symptoms often need to be in the hospital. They will be given fluids in a vein and airway support.
- There is not yet a vaccine to prevent WNV in humans.

❺ West Nile Virus Spread by Mosquitoes

- West Nile virus is spread by the bite of a mosquito. The mosquito gets the virus from biting infected birds.
- Even in an area where the virus occurs, less than 1% of mosquitoes carry it.
- Spread is mosquito to human.

- Person-to-person spread does not occur. Kissing, touching, or sharing a glass with a person who has WNV is safe.

- Mothers with mosquito bites can breastfeed (Centers for Disease Control and Prevention 2003) unless they get symptoms of the virus.

- It takes 3 to 14 days after the mosquito bite to get the virus.

- In the United States and Canada, peak summers for WNV were 2002, 2003, and 2012.

Insect Repellent Questions

❶ Prevention Tips

- Wear long pants, a long-sleeved shirt, and a hat.

- Avoid being outside when bugs are most active. Mosquitoes are most active at dawn and dusk. Limit your child's outdoor play during these times.

- Get rid of any standing water. (**Reason:** It's where they lay their eggs.)

- Keep bugs out of your home by fixing any broken screens.

- Insect repellents containing DEET are very good at preventing mosquito bites. Read the label carefully.

❷ DEET Products: Use on the Skin

- DEET is a good mosquito repellent. It also repels ticks and other bugs.

- The American Academy of Pediatrics approves DEET use for infants and children older than 2 months. Use 30% DEET or less. Use 30% DEET if you need 6 hours of protection. Use 10% DEET if you need protection for only 2 hours.

- Don't put DEET on the hands if your child sucks his thumb or fingers. (**Reason:** Prevents swallowing DEET.)

- Warn older children who apply their own DEET to use less. A total of 3 or 4 drops can protect the whole body.

- Put on exposed areas of the skin. Do not use near the eyes or mouth. Don't use on skin that is covered by clothing. Don't put DEET on sunburns or rashes. (**Reason:** DEET can be easily absorbed in these areas.)

- Wash it off with soap and water when your child comes indoors.

- **Caution:** DEET can damage clothing made of manmade fibers. It can also damage plastics (eyeglasses) and leather. DEET can be used on cotton clothing.

❸ Permethrin Product: Use on Clothing

- Products that contain permethrin (such as Duranon) work well to repel mosquitos and ticks.
- Unlike DEET, these products are put on clothing instead of skin.
- Put it on shirt or pant cuffs, shoes, and hats. Can also put it on mosquito nets and sleeping bags.
- Do not put permethrin on the skin. (**Reason:** Sweat changes it so it does not work.)

❹ Picaridin Products

- Picaridin is a repellent that is equal to 10% DEET.
- It can safely be put on skin or clothing.

Remember!
Contact your doctor if your child develops any of the **Call Your Doctor** symptoms.

CHAPTER 55

Tick Bite

Definition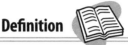

- A tick (small brown bug) is attached to the skin.
- A tick was removed from the skin.

Symptoms of a Tick Bite

- A tick bite does not usually cause pain or itch. So, ticks may not be noticed for a few days.
- After feeding on blood, a tick gets swollen and easier to see.
- Ticks fall off on their own after sucking blood for 3 to 6 days.
- After the tick comes off, a little red bump may be seen.
- The red bump or spot is the body's response to the tick's saliva (spit).
- While it's sucking blood, some of its saliva gets mixed in.

Causes of Tick Bites

- A wood (dog) tick is the size of an apple seed. After feeding, it can double or triple in size. Sometimes, it can pass on Rocky Mountain spotted fever or Colorado tick fever.
- A deer tick is the size of a poppy seed. After feeding, it can triple in size. Sometimes, it can pass on Lyme disease.

Lyme Disease

- More than 95% of people who get Lyme disease live in or have traveled to 14 high-risk states. Lyme disease occurs mainly in the Northeast, mid-Atlantic, and upper Midwest. Many states do not have Lyme disease. The Centers for Disease Control and Prevention reports more than 30,000 new cases per year (2020).
- About 80% of Lyme disease starts with a bull's-eye rash called *erythema migrans*. The rash starts at the site of the tick bite. It starts on the average at 7 days. It

grows larger quickly, to more than 2 in (5 cm) wide. It can become as large as 12 in (30 cm). It lasts 2 or 3 weeks. Treatment of this rash with an antibiotic is advised. This almost always prevents later stages of Lyme disease. If Lyme disease isn't treated, heart, joint, and neurologic problems can occur.

▶ Giving antibiotics after deer tick bites to prevent Lyme disease depends on the risk. The risk is low with brief attachment. The risk is high if the deer tick was attached for longer than 36 hours. It's also higher if the tick is swollen, not flat. Ask your doctor for advice.

▶ Risk of Lyme disease after a deer tick bite is low. But, in high-risk areas, 2% of deer tick bites causes Lyme disease.

When to Call Your Doctor

Call Your Doctor Now (Night or Day) If

▶ Can't remove the tick after trying this chapter's Care Advice.

▶ Widespread rash starts 2 to 14 days after the bite.

▶ Fever or headache starts 2 to 14 days after the bite.

▶ Fever and bite looks infected (spreading redness).

▶ Weak, droopy eyelid, droopy face, or crooked smile.

▶ Your child looks or acts very sick.

▶ You think your child needs to be seen, and the problem is urgent.

Call Your Doctor Within 24 Hours If

▶ Deer tick was attached for more than 36 hours.

▶ Deer tick is swollen, not flat.

▶ New redness starts more than 24 hours after the bite. (**Note:** Bacterial infection is rare. It does not start until at least 24–48 hours after the bite.)

▶ More than 48 hours since the bite and red area now getting larger.

▶ Red-ring or bull's-eye rash occurs around a deer tick bite. (**Note:** The rash of Lyme disease starts 3–30 days after the bite.)

▶ You think your child needs to be seen, but the problem is not urgent.

Call Your Doctor During Weekday Office Hours If

▶ You have other questions or concerns.

Parent Care at Home If

▶ Tick bite with no complications.

▶ Preventing tick bites.

Care Advice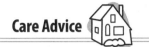

Treating Tick Bites

❶ What You Should Know About Wood Tick Bites

- Most wood tick bites are harmless.

- Spread of disease by wood ticks is not common.

- If the tick is still attached to the skin, it needs to be taken off.

- Try one of the methods described below to take out the tick.

❷ Wood Tick: How to Remove It With Tweezers

- Use tweezers. Grasp the tick as close to the skin as possible (on its head).

- Hold the tweezers sideways next to the top of the skin.

- Pull the wood tick straight upward without twisting or crushing it.

- Keep a steady pressure until the tick lets go of its grip.

- If you don't have tweezers, you can use your fingers.

- **Other options:** You can use a loop of thread around the jaws. You can also use a needle pushed between the jaws for traction. Jaws are the part of the head attached to the skin.

- **Caution:** Covering the tick with petroleum jelly or nail polish doesn't work. Neither does rubbing alcohol or a soapy cotton ball. Touching the tick with a hot or cold object also doesn't work.

❸ What You Should Know About Deer Tick Bites

- Most deer tick bites are harmless.

- The spread of disease by deer ticks is not common.

- Even in high-risk areas, only 2% of deer tick bites cause Lyme disease.

- Most people who get Lyme disease live in or have traveled to 14 high-risk states. Lyme disease occurs mainly in the Northeast and upper Midwest. Many states do not have Lyme disease.

❹ Deer Tick: How to Remove It

- If it is swollen, try to remove with tweezers. (See number 2 of this advice.)
- Tiny deer ticks need to be scraped off.
- You can remove them with the edge of a credit card.

❺ Tick's Head: How to Remove It

- If the wood tick's head (mouth parts) breaks off in the skin, remove any large pieces.
- Clean the skin with rubbing alcohol.
- Use clean tweezers or a clean needle to scrape it off.
- If a small piece remains, the skin will slowly heal and shed it.

❻ Antibiotic Ointment

- After the tick is removed, wash the wound with soap and water. Also, wash your hands after you are done.
- This helps prevent catching any infections carried by the tick.
- Use an antibiotic ointment (such as Polysporin). No prescription is needed.
- Put it on the bite once.

❼ What to Expect

- Most often, tick bites don't usually itch or hurt.
- That's why they may not be noticed.
- The little bump goes away in 2 days.
- If the tick transferred a disease, a rash will occur. It will appear in the next 4 weeks.

❽ Call Your Doctor If

- You tried and can't remove the tick.
- Fever or rash happens in the next 4 weeks.
- Bite starts to look infected.
- You think your child needs to be seen.
- Your child becomes worse.

Prevent Tick Bites

❶ Prevent Tick Bites

- After being outdoors in deer tick areas, check for ticks. Remove any that are attached. Also, take a shower soon after coming inside.

- Tumble dry any clothing in a hot dryer for 10 minutes. That should kill any ticks left in clothing.

- When hiking outside where there are ticks, wear long clothing. Tuck the ends of pants into socks. Use a bug repellent on shoes, socks, and exposed skin.

❷ Tick Repellent for Clothing: Permethrin

- Permethrin products (such as Duranon) work well to repel ticks.

- Unlike DEET, these products are put on clothing instead of skin. They also can last through many washes. Use them on pant cuffs, socks, and shoes. You can also put them on other outdoor items (bug netting, sleeping bags).

- Do not put permethrin on skin. (**Reason:** Sweat changes it so it does not work.)

❸ Tick Repellent for Skin: DEET

- DEET also works well to repel ticks. It can be used on the skin not covered by clothing.

- Use 30% DEET for children and teens (American Academy of Pediatrics). **Note:** 30% DEET protects for 6 hours.

- DEET is approved for use in infants and children older than 2 months (American Academy of Pediatrics).

Remember!
Contact your doctor if your child develops any of the **Call Your Doctor** symptoms.

PART 14

Miscellaneous Symptoms

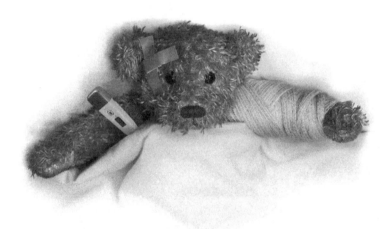

CHAPTER 56

Emergency Symptoms Not to Miss

Most life-threatening emergencies are easy to recognize. You would not overlook major bleeding, breathing that stops, a seizure, or a coma. You would call **911** for help. If you suspected poisoning, you would call the Poison Help Line at **1-800-222-1222**. Some emergency symptoms, however, can be missed or ignored. See the following list of symptoms. If your child has any of these symptoms, call your child's doctor now. If you can't reach your child's doctor, go to the nearest ER. For a few of these symptoms, call 911. Some emergency symptoms, however, can be missed or ignored. Here's that important list.

Sick Newborn

▸ Your baby is younger than 1 month and has a fever or looks sick. This includes vomiting, cough, or even poor color. Your baby may start to act abnormal if she is getting sick. Examples are poor feeding or sleeping too much. At this age, these symptoms are serious until proven otherwise. During the first month of life, infections can progress very fast.

Lethargy

▸ Your young child is lethargic if she stares into space or won't smile. She won't play at all or hardly responds to you. Your child is too weak to cry or hard to wake up. These are serious symptoms.

▸ **Note:** Sleeping more when sick is normal. When awake, your child should be alert.

Confusion

▸ Sudden onset of confusion is serious. Your child is awake but says strange things. She sees things that aren't there. She doesn't recognize you.

▸ **Note:** Brief confusion for 5 minutes or so can be seen with high fevers. This can be normal. But if not brief, confusion can have some serious causes.

Severe Pain

▸ Severe pain keeps your child from doing all normal activities. Your child won't play or even watch a favorite TV show. She just wants to be left alone. Your child may cry when you try to hold or move her. Children with severe pain also can't sleep or can fall asleep only briefly.

Inconsolable Crying

▸ Inconsolable, constant crying is caused by severe pain until proven otherwise. Suspect this in children who can't sleep or can fall asleep only briefly. When awake, they will not join in any normal activities. They won't play or may be distracted. They may be very hard to console. (**Caution:** Instead of crying, severe pain may cause your child to moan or whimper.)

Can't Walk

▸ If your child has learned to walk and then suddenly won't, call your doctor. She may have a serious injury to the legs or a problem with balance. If your child walks bent over holding her stomach, she may have appendicitis.

Vomits Bile

▸ Vomiting that is bright green is most often bile. Unless your child drank a green liquid, this is not normal. It can mean the intestines are blocked up. This is a surgical emergency.

▸ **Note:** Vomiting some yellow fluid is normal. The yellow color is from stomach acid.

Tender Belly

▸ Press on your child's belly while she is distracted by a toy or book. You should be able to press in 1 in (2.5 cm) or so without a problem. If your child winces or screams, it suggests a serious cause. If the belly is also bloated and hard, the problem is more urgent.

▸ **Note:** If your child just pushes your hand away, you haven't distracted her enough.

Pain in Testicle or Scrotum

▶ Sudden pain in the scrotum can be from twisting (torsion) of the testicle. This needs surgery within 8 hours to save the testicle.

Trouble Breathing

▶ Breathing is essential for life. Most childhood deaths are caused by severe breathing problems. Breathing problems can be caused by throat or lung infections. Parents need to learn to recognize trouble breathing. If your child has tight croup or wheezing, she needs to be seen now. Other bad signs are fast breathing, grunting with each breath, bluish lips, or retractions. This means the skin pulls in between the ribs with each breath. It is a sign of trouble breathing in younger children. Children with severe breathing problems can't drink, talk, or cry. If your child is struggling to breathe, call 911.

Bluish or Gray Lips

▶ Bluish or gray lips, tongue, or gums can mean not enough oxygen in the bloodstream. Call 911.

▶ **Note:** Bluish skin around only the mouth (not the lips) can be normal. It can be caused by being cold or afraid.

Trouble Swallowing With Drooling

▶ Sudden onset of drooling or spitting means your child is having trouble swallowing. Most often, this is from severe swelling in the throat. The cause can be a serious throat infection. A serious allergic reaction can also cause trouble swallowing. Swelling in the throat could close off the airway.

Dehydration

► Dehydration means your child's body fluids are low. Dehydration is often caused by severe vomiting or diarrhea. Suspect dehydration if your child has not urinated in 8 hours. Crying no tears and a dry inside of the mouth (tongue) are also signs. In young babies, the soft spot in the head is sunken. Dehydrated children are also tired and weak.

► **Note:** If your child is alert, playful, and active, she is not yet dehydrated. Children with severe dehydration become dizzy when they stand. Dehydration needs extra fluids by mouth or vein.

Bulging Soft Spot

► The soft spot in your baby's head is tense and bulging. This means the brain is under pressure.

Stiff Neck

► A stiff neck means your child can't touch chin to chest. To test for a stiff neck, lay your child down. Then lift her head until the chin touches the chest. If she fights you, place a toy or coin on the belly. This makes her have to look down to see it. Older children can simply be asked to look at their belly button. A stiff neck can be an early sign of meningitis.

► **Note:** Without fever, a stiff neck is often from sore neck muscles.

Neck Injury

► Talk with your child's doctor about any neck injury, regardless of symptoms. Neck injuries carry a risk of damage to the spinal cord.

Purple or Blood-Red Spots or Dots

- ▶ Purple or blood-red spots or dots on the skin need to be seen. When present with fever, they could be a sign of a serious bloodstream infection. The color of these serious rashes will not change when you press on them. The color of normal viral rashes will fade with skin pressure.

- ▶ **Note:** Bumps and bruises on the shins from active play are different.

Fever (Above 100.4°F or 38°C) in the First 3 Months

- ▶ Fevers in newborns and young babies are treated differently than fevers in older children. Bacterial infections are more common at this age and can worsen quickly. A fever is a rectal or forehead temperature of 100.4°F (38°C) or higher. All babies younger than 3 months with a fever need to be seen now. They need tests to decide if the cause is viral or bacterial.

Fever Above 105°F (40.6°C)

- ▶ A fever tells you your child has an infection. Serious infections can occur with low-grade fevers as well as higher fevers. All the above symptoms are stronger signs of serious illness than the level of fever. Research shows fevers alone are a risk factor only when very high. That means levels above 105°F (40.6°C). So, call your doctor if your child's fever goes above 104°F (40°C). This is a safe rule.

Chronic Diseases

- ▶ Most active chronic diseases can have some serious complications. If your child has a chronic disease, learn what those complications are. Find out how to recognize early changes. Diseases at highest risk for serious infections are those that weaken the immune system. These include sickle cell disease, HIV, cancer, organ transplant, or taking oral steroids. If you are talking with health care professionals who don't know your child, speak up. Always tell them about your child's chronic disease (such as asthma). Never assume doctors and nurses already know this.

CHAPTER 57

Immunization Reactions

Definition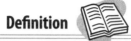

▶ Reactions to a recent immunization (vaccine).

• Most are reactions at the shot site (such as pain, swelling, or redness).

• General reactions (such as a fever or being fussy) may also occur.

▶ Reactions to the following vaccines are covered:

• Chickenpox (varicella) virus.

• COVID-19 virus.

• DTaP (diphtheria, tetanus, and pertussis).

• *Haemophilus influenzae* type b.

• Hepatitis A virus.

• Hepatitis B virus.

• Human papillomavirus.

• Influenza virus.

• MMR (measles-mumps-rubella).

• Meningococcal.

• Polio virus.

• Pneumococcal.

• Rotavirus.

• Tuberculosis (TB) (BCG vaccine).

Symptoms of Vaccine Reactions

▶ **Local reactions.** Shot sites can have swelling, redness, and pain. Most often, these symptoms start within 24 hours of the shot and last 3 to 5 days. With the DTaP vaccine, they can last up to 7 days.

▶ **Fever.** Fever with most vaccines begins within 24 hours and lasts 1 to 2 days.

- **Delayed reactions.** With the MMR and chickenpox shots, fever and rash can occur. These symptoms start later. They usually begin between 1 and 4 weeks.

- **Anaphylaxis.** Severe allergic reactions are very rare. They start within 20 minutes. Sometimes, they can occur up to 2 hours after the shot. Vaccine site nurses know how to treat these reactions.

Vaccine App

- Vaccines on the Go is a free app from Children's Hospital of Philadelphia (CHOP).

- This app can answer any vaccine question you might have.

- It is fact based and up to date.

When to Call Your Doctor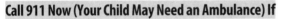

Call 911 Now (Your Child May Need an Ambulance) If

- Trouble breathing or swallowing.

- Not moving or very weak.

- Can't wake up.

- You think your child has a life-threatening emergency.

Go to ER Now If

- Hard to wake up.

Call Your Doctor Now (Night or Day) If

- Younger than 12 weeks with fever. (**Caution:** Do *not* give your baby any fever medicine before being seen.)

- Fever above 104°F (40°C).

- Fever after vaccine given and weak immune system (such as sickle cell disease, HIV, cancer, organ transplant, or taking oral steroids).

- High-pitched crying lasts more than 1 hour.

- Nonstop crying lasts more than 3 hours.

- Rotavirus vaccine followed by vomiting or severe crying.

- Your child looks or acts very sick.

- You think your child needs to be seen, and the problem is urgent.

Call Your Doctor Within 24 Hours If

▸ Redness or red streak starts more than 48 hours (2 days) after the shot.

▸ Redness around the shot becomes larger than 3 in (7.6 cm).

▸ Fever lasts more than 3 days.

▸ Fever returns after being gone for more than 24 hours.

▸ Measles vaccine rash (which starts day 6–12 after the shot) lasts more than 4 days.

▸ You think your child needs to be seen, but the problem is not urgent.

Call Your Doctor During Weekday Office Hours If

▸ Redness or red streak around the shot is larger than 1 in (2.5 cm).

▸ Redness, swelling, or pain is getting worse after 3 days.

▸ Fussiness from vaccine lasts more than 3 days.

▸ You have other questions or concerns.

Parent Care at Home If

▸ Normal immunization reaction.

Care Advice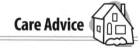

Treatment for Common Immunization Reactions

❶ What You Should Know About Common Shot Reactions

- Immunizations (vaccines) protect your child against serious diseases.

- Pain, redness, and swelling are normal where the shot was given. Most symptoms start within the first 12 hours after the shot was given. Redness and fever starting on day 1 of the shot are always normal.

- All of these reactions mean the vaccine is working.

- Your child's body is making new antibodies to protect against the real disease.

- Most of these symptoms will last only 2 or 3 days.

- There is no need to see your doctor for normal reactions, such as redness or fever.

- Here is some care advice that should help.

❷ Vaccine Injection Site Reaction: Treatment

- Some pain, swelling, and skin redness at the injection site is normal. It means the vaccine is working.

- **Massage:** Gently massage the injection site 3 or more times a day.

- **Heat:** For pain or redness, apply a heating pad or a warm, wet washcloth to the area for 10 minutes. Repeat as needed. (**Reason:** Will increase blood flow to the area. May apply cold if you prefer, but avoid ice.)

- **No pain medicine:** Try not to give any pain medicines. (**Reason:** Pain medicines may reduce the body's normal immune response.) Use local heat instead. Pain rarely worsens.

- **Hives at the shot site:** If itchy, can put on 1% hydrocortisone cream (such as Cortaid). No prescription is needed. Use twice daily as needed.

❸ Fever With Vaccines: Treatment

- Fever with vaccines is normal, harmless, and probably beneficial. (**Reason:** Fever speeds up your body's immune system.)

- Fever with most vaccines begins within 12 hours and lasts 1 to 2 days.

- For low-grade fevers, 100°F to 102°F (37.8°C–39°C), do not give fever medicines. (**Reason:** They may reduce your body's normal immune response.)

- For fevers above 102°F (39°C), medicine may be given for discomfort. If needed, use acetaminophen. (See drug dosage chart in the Appendix.)

- **Fluids.** Encourage cool fluids in unlimited amounts. (**Reason:** Prevents dehydration.) Fluids can also lower high fevers. If younger than 6 months, only give formula or breast milk.

- **Clothing.** Dress in normal clothing. For shivering or the chills, use a blanket until it stops.

❹ General Symptoms From Vaccines

- All vaccines can cause mild fussiness, crying, and restless sleep. This is usually due to a sore shot site.

- Some children sleep more than usual. A decreased appetite and activity level are also common.

- These symptoms are normal. They do not need any treatment.

- They will usually go away within 24 to 48 hours.

❺ Call Your Doctor If

- Redness starts after 2 days (48 hours).
- Redness becomes larger than 2 in (5.1 cm).
- Pain or redness worsens after 3 days (or lasts more than 7 days).
- Fever starts after 2 days (or lasts more than 3 days).
- You think your child needs to be seen.
- Your child becomes worse.

Specific Immunization Reactions

❶ Chickenpox (Varicella) Virus Vaccine

- Pain or swelling at the shot site for 1 to 2 days (20% of children).
- Mild fever lasting 1 to 3 days begins 14 to 28 days after the shot (10%). Give acetaminophen or ibuprofen for fever above 102°F (39°C).
- Never give aspirin for fever, for pain, or within 6 weeks of getting the shot. (**Reason:** Risk of Reye syndrome, a rare but serious brain disease.)
- Chickenpox-like rash (usually 2 red bumps) at the shot site (3%).
- Chickenpox-like rash (usually 5 red bumps) scattered over the body (4%).
- This mild rash begins 5 to 26 days after the shot. Most often, it lasts a few days.
- Children with these rashes can go to child care or school. (**Reason:** For practical purposes, vaccine rashes are not spread to others.)
- **Exception:** Do not go to school if red bumps drain fluid and are widespread. (**Reason:** Can be actual chickenpox.)
- **Caution:** If vaccine rash contains fluid, cover it with clothing. You can also use a bandage (such as a Band-Aid).

❷ COVID-19 Virus Vaccine

- **Injection site reactions.** Pain and tenderness start within 8 hours (90% of patients). Other local reactions are some swelling (10%) or skin redness (5%). Local symptoms usually last 1 to 3 days.
- **General body symptoms.** Fever (15%), chills (40%), tiredness (70%), muscle aches (50%), and headaches (60%). General symptoms start at about 24 hours. They usually last 1 day, sometimes 2.
- **Vaccines with 2 doses.** Symptoms are more frequent after the second vaccine. The previous symptoms are for the second dose.

- **Vaccines with 1 dose.** Side effects were the same type but a little less frequent.
- The vaccine does not cause any respiratory symptoms such as cough, runny nose, or shortness of breath.
- It is impossible to get COVID-19 from the vaccine. (**Reason:** There is no live COVID-19 virus in the vaccine.)
- Severe allergic reactions to the vaccine are very rare.

❸ DTaP (Diphtheria, Tetanus, and Pertussis) Vaccine

- The following harmless reactions to DTaP can occur:
  - Pain, tenderness, swelling, and redness at the shot site are the main side effects. This happens in 25% of children. It usually starts within the first 12 hours. Redness and fever starting on day 1 of the shot are always normal. They last for 3 to 7 days.
  - Fever (in 25% of children) and lasts for 24 to 48 hours.
  - Mild drowsiness (30%), fretfulness (30%), or poor appetite (10%) and lasts for 24 to 48 hours.
  - Large swelling over 4 in (10.2 cm) can follow later doses of DTaP. The area of redness is smaller. This usually occurs with the fourth or fifth dose. It occurs in 5% of children. Most children can still move the leg or arm normally, but may walk with a limp.
  - The large thigh or upper arm swelling goes away without treatment by day 3 (60%) to day 7 (90%).
  - This is not an allergy. Future DTaP vaccines are safe to give.

❹ *Haemophilus influenzae* Type B Vaccine

- No serious reactions reported.
- Sore injection site or mild fever occurs in only 2% of children.

❺ Hepatitis A Virus Vaccine

- No serious reactions reported.
- Sore injection occurs in 20% of children.
- Loss of appetite occurs in 10% of children.
- Headache occurs in 5% of children.
- Most often, no fever is present.
- If these symptoms occur, they most often last 1 to 2 days.

❻ Hepatitis B Virus Vaccine

■ No serious reactions reported.

■ Sore shot site occurs in 30% of children and mild fever in 3% of children.

■ Fever from the vaccine is rare. Any baby younger than 2 months with a fever after this shot should be examined.

❼ Human Papillomavirus Vaccine

■ No serious reactions.

■ Sore injection site for few days in 90% of children.

■ Mild redness and swelling at the shot site (in 50%).

■ Fever above 100.4°F (38°C) in 10% and fever above 102°F (39°C) in 2%.

■ Headache in 30%.

❽ Influenza Virus Vaccine

■ Pain, tenderness, or swelling at the injection site occurs within 6 to 8 hours. This happens in 10% of children.

■ Mild fever below 103°F (39.5°C) occurs in 20% of children. Fevers occur mainly in young children.

■ **Nasal influenza vaccine:** Congested or runny nose and mild fever.

❾ Measles Vaccine (Part of MMR)

■ The measles shot can cause a fever (in 10% of children) and rash (in 5% of children). This occurs about 6 to 12 days after the shot.

■ Mild fever below 103°F (39.5°C) in 10% and lasts 2 or 3 days.

■ The mild pink rash is mainly on the trunk and lasts 2 or 3 days.

■ No treatment is needed. The rash cannot be spread to others. Your child can go to child care or to school with the rash.

■ **Call your doctor if**

– Rash changes to blood-colored spots.

– Rash lasts more than 3 days.

❿ Mumps-Rubella (Part of MMR)

■ There are no serious reactions.

■ Sometimes, a sore shot site can occur.

⑪ Meningococcal Vaccine

- No serious reactions.
- Sore shot site for 1 to 2 days occurs in 50% of children. Limited use of the arm occurs in 15%.
- Mild fever occurs in 5%; headache, in 40%; and joint pain, in 20%.
- The vaccine never causes meningitis.

⑫ Polio Virus Vaccine

- Polio vaccine given by shot sometimes causes some muscle soreness.
- Polio vaccine given by mouth is no longer used in the United States.

⑬ Pneumococcal Vaccine

- No serious reactions.
- Pain, tenderness, swelling, or redness at the injection site in 20%.
- Mild fever below 102°F (39°C) in 15% for 1 to 2 days.

⑭ Rotavirus Vaccine

- Most often, no serious reactions to this vaccine given by mouth.
- Mild diarrhea or vomiting for 1 to 2 days in 3% of children.
- No fever.
- Rare serious reaction: intussusception risk in 1 in 100,000 (Centers for Disease Control and Prevention). Presents with vomiting or severe crying.

⑮ BCG Vaccine for Tuberculosis (TB)

- Vaccine used to prevent TB in high-risk groups or countries. It is not used in the United States or most of Canada. (**Note:** This is different than the skin test placed on the forearm to detect TB.)
- BCG vaccine is given into the skin of the right shoulder area.
- Timing: Mainly given to infants and young children.
- **Normal reaction:** After 6 to 8 weeks, a blister forms. It gradually enlarges and eventually drains a whitish yellow liquid. The blister then heals, leaving a scar. The raised scar is proof of BCG protection against TB.
- **Abnormal reaction:** Abscess (infected lump) occurs in the shoulder or under the arm. Occurs in 1% of patients.

■ **Call your doctor if**

- Blister turns into a large red lump.

- Lymph node in the armpit becomes large.

Remember!

Contact your doctor if your child develops any of the **Call Your Doctor** symptoms.

Drug Dosage Charts

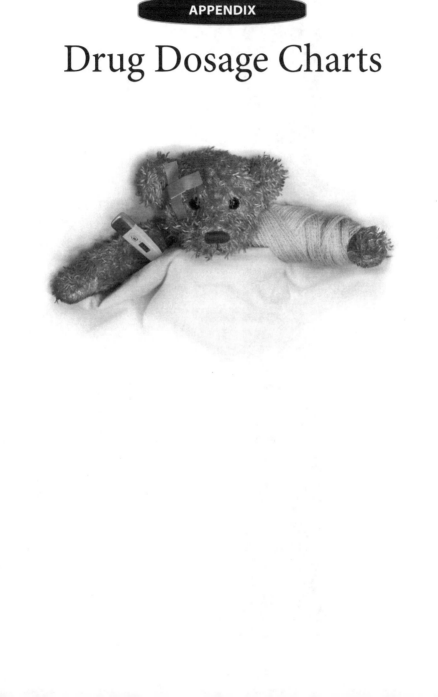

352
My Child Is Sick!

Acetaminophen Dosage Chart: Medicine for Pain or Fever, Such as Tylenol

Medicine Product	Child's Weight (Pounds)								
	6–11 lb	12–17 lb	18–23 lb	24–35 lb	36–47 lb	48–59 lb	60–71 lb	72–95 lb	96+ lb
Infant Liquid 160 mg/5 mL	1.25 mL	2.5 mL	3.75 mL	5 mL					
Children's Liquid 160 mg/5 mL	1.25 mL	2.5 mL	3.75 mL	5 mL	7.5 mL	10 mL	12.5 mL	15 mL	20 mL
Children's Chewable Junior 160-mg tablets				1	1½	2	2½	3	4
Adult Regular-strength 325-mg tablets						1	1	1½	2
Adult Extra-strength 500-mg tablets								1	1

Chart Notes

- **Brand Name:** Tylenol or store brand.

- **Dose:** Find your child's weight (lb) in the top row of the dose chart. Look below the correct weight for the dose based on the product you have.
    - Adult Dose: 500 to 650 mg
    - Adult Daily Maximum: 3,000 mg in 24 hours

- **Measure the Dose:** Use the syringe or dropper that comes with the medicine. If not, you can buy a medicine syringe at a drugstore. If you use a teaspoon, it must be a measuring spoon. **Reason:** Regular spoons are not reliable. **Keep in Mind:** 1 level teaspoon equals 5 mL (mL stands for milliliter).

- **How Often:** Repeat every 4 to 6 hours as needed. Don't give more than 5 times a day.

- **Age Limit:** Don't use younger than 12 weeks unless told to by your child's doctor. **Reason:** For any fever in the first 12 weeks of life, your baby needs to be seen now.

- **Caution:** Do not use acetaminophen and ibuprofen together. **Reason:** No benefit over using one medicine alone and a risk of giving too much. **Exception:** Your child's doctor told you to give both.

Ibuprofen Dosage Chart: Medicine for Pain or Fever, Such as Advil or Motrin

Medicine Product	Child's Weight (Pounds)							
	12–17 lb	18–23 lb	24–35 lb	36–47 lb	48–59 lb	60–71 lb	72–95 lb	96+ lb
Infant Liquid 50 mg/1.25 mL	1.25 mL	1.875 mL	2.5 mL	3.75 mL				
Children's Liquid 100 mg/5 mL			5 mL	7.5 mL	10 mL	12.5 mL	15 mL	20 mL
Children's Chewable 100-mg tablets			1	1½	2	2½	3	4
Children's 100-mg tablets					2	2	3	4
Adult 200-mg tablets					1	1	1½	2

Chart Notes

- **Brand Names:** Advil, Motrin, or store brand.

- **Dose:** Find your child's weight (lb) in the top row of the dose chart. Look below the correct weight for the dose based on the product you have. Adult dose is 400 mg.
  - Adult Dose: 400 mg
  - Adult Daily Maximum: 1,200 mg in 24 hours (unless directed by a health care provider)

- **Measure the Dose:** Use the syringe or dropper that comes with the medicine. If not, you can buy a medicine syringe at a drugstore. If you use a teaspoon, it must be a measuring spoon. **Reason:** Regular spoons are not reliable. **Keep in Mind:** 1 level teaspoon equals 5 mL (mL stands for milliliter).

- **How Often:** Repeat every 6 to 8 hours as needed. Don't give more than 3 times a day.

- **Age Limit:** Don't use younger than 6 months unless told to by your child's doctor. **Reason:** For any fever in the first 12 weeks of life, your baby needs to be seen now. Also, the FDA has not approved ibuprofen for infants younger than 6 months.

- **Caution:** Do not use acetaminophen and ibuprofen together. **Reason:** No benefit over using one medicine alone and a risk of giving too much. **Exception:** Your child's doctor told you to give both.

Benadryl Dosage Chart (Diphenhydramine): Medicine for Allergies or Hives

Medicine Product	Child's Weight (Pounds)					
	20–24 lb	25–37 lb	38–49 lb	50–99 lb	100+ lb
Liquid 12.5 mg/5 mL	4 mL	5 mL	7.5 mL	10 mL	
Chewable 12.5-mg tablets		1	1½	2	4
Adult 25-mg tablets		½	½	1	2
Adult 25-mg capsules				1	2

Chart Notes

Brand Names: Benadryl or store brand. Use an allergy product that has just one medicine in it. Avoid allergy medicines that also treat nose congestion.

Dose: Find you child's weight (lb) in the top row of the dosage chart. Look below the correct weight for the dose based on the product you have. Adult dose is 50 mg.

Measure the Dose: Use the syringe that comes with the medicine. If not, you can buy a medicine syringe at a drugstore. If you use a teaspoon, it must be a measuring spoon. **Reason:** Regular spoons are not reliable. **Keep in Mind:** 1 level teaspoon equals 5 mL (mL stands for milliliter).

How Often: Repeat every 6 to 8 hours as needed.

Age Limit: For allergies, don't use younger than 1 year unless told to by your child's doctor. **Reason:** It causes most babies to be sleepy. For colds, not advised at any age. **Reason:** No proven benefits.

Reviewers

The author is grateful to the following individuals for their time and expertise in reviewing some of the pediatric clinical content that has been incorporated into these guidelines:

Medical Directors of Pediatric Call Centers
Peter Dehnel, MD, Children's Physician Network, Minneapolis, MN
Andrew Hertz, MD, Rainbow Babies Children's Hospital, Cleveland, OH
Susan MacLean, MD, Sykes Assistance Services Corporation, Toronto, Ontario, Canada
Dan Nicklas, MD, Children's Hospital Colorado, Aurora, CO
Peter O'Hanley, MD, Sykes Assistance Services Corporation, Moncton, New Brunswick, Canada
Randy Sterkel, MD, St. Louis Children's Hospital, St Louis, MO
Debra Weiner, MD, Citra Health, Portland, ME (former)
Elaine Donoghue, MD, St. Peter's Medical Center Call Center, New Brunswick, NJ (former)
Hanna Sherman, MD, Boston Children's Hospital Call Center, Boston, MA (former)

Pediatric Emergency Medicine Specialists
Lalit Bajaj, MD, Children's Hospital Colorado
Joan Bothner, MD, Children's Hospital Colorado
Alison Brent, MD, Children's Hospital Colorado
Michael DiStefano, MD, Children's Hospital Colorado
Cinnamon Dixon, DO, Children's Hospital Colorado
Joseph Grubenhoff, MD, Children's Hospital Colorado

Community Pediatrician Advisory Board: Children's Hospital Colorado, Aurora, CO
Vincent DiMaria, MD, Arapahoe Park Pediatrics, Littleton, CO
Matt Dorighi, MD, Cherry Creek Pediatrics, Denver, CO
John Guenther MD, Fort Collins Youth Clinic, Fort Collins, CO
Daniel Feiten, MD, Greenwood Pediatrics, Centennial, CO
Michael Kurtz, MD, Advanced Pediatric Associates, Aurora, CO
Jay Markson, MD, Children's Medical Center, Denver, CO
Robert Mauro, MD, Greenwood Pediatrics, Littleton, CO
Martha Middlemist, MD, Pediatrics at 5280, Englewood, CO
Michelle Stanford, MD, Centennial Pediatrics, Centennial, CO
Stephanie Stevens, MD, Advanced Pediatric Associates, Aurora, CO

Community Pediatrician Advisory Board: St. Louis Children's Hospital, St Louis, MO
Tara Copper, MD, Emergency Medicine, Washington University SOM
Jay Epstein, MD, Community Pediatrician, Forest Park Pediatrics
Robert Kebler, MD, Community Pediatrician, Suburban Pediatrics
Steve Lillpop, MD, Community Pediatrician, Jacksonville Pediatrics
Mark Lowe, MD, Pediatrics Department Administration, Washington University
SOM
Jerome O'Neil, MD, Community Pediatrician, Southwest Pediatrics
Rachel Orscheln, MD, Infectious Disease, Washington University SOM
Casey Pruitt, MD, Complex Care Pediatrician, Academic Pediatrics, Washington
University SOM
Isabel Rosenbloom, MD, Community Pediatrician, Tots Thru Teens Pediatrics
Harold Sitrin, MD, Community Pediatrician, Suburban Pediatrics
David Sonderman, MD, Community Pediatrician, Children's Clinic
Kristin Stahl, MD, Community Pediatrician, Heartland Pediatrics
Randy Sterkel, MD, Answer Line Medical Director, Community Pediatrician, Esse
Health Pediatrics
Mary Tillman, MD, Community Pediatrician, Tillman Pediatrics

Telephone Triage Nurses: Pediatric Call Center, Children's Hospital Colorado, Aurora, CO
Teresa Baird, RN
Jenn Engel, RN
Teresa Hegarty, RN
Kelly Hering-Rank, RN
Liz Lindvall, RN
Kathleen Martinez, RN
Kelli Massaro, RN
Julie Munder, RN
Sara Nudd, RN
Deanna Miller, RN
Nicole Thede, RN, PNP

Telephone Triage Nurses: Other Sites
Audra Bailey, RN, Aurora, CO
Amy Barrett, RN, Portland, OR
Jacquie Berry, RN, Minnetonka, MN
Charlene Brophy, RN, Newfoundland, Canada
Jeanine Feirer, RN, Unity, WI
Bev Hansen, RN, Philadelphia, PA
Laticia Humphrey, RN, Knoxville, TN
Wanda Janes, RN, Newfoundland, Canada

Lori Leaf, RN, Alberta, Canada
Melissa Masson, RN, London, Ontario, Canada
Cheryl Patterson, RN, Evergreen, WA
Michelle Ramey, RN, Fort Worth, TX
Ann Schauer, RN, Sioux City, IA
Meghan Senior, RN, St Louis, MO
Lisa Swerczek, RN, St Louis, MO

Pediatric Subspecialists: Children's Hospital Colorado, Aurora, CO *(Unless Otherwise Noted)*
Adolescent Medicine: David Kaplan, MD; Eric Sigel, MD; Karolyn Kabir, MD;
   Molly Richards, MD (Family Planning); and Amy Sass, MD
Allergy: Dan Atkins, MD, and James Shira, MD
Behavior: Kimberly Kelsay, MD, and Ayelet Talmi, PhD
Breastfeeding: Maya Bunik, MD
Cardiology: Michael Schaffer, MD; Robert Wolfe, MD; and Henry Sondheimer, MD
Child Abuse: Andrew Sirotnak, MD, and Antonia Chiesa, MD
Dentistry: Elizabeth A. Shick, DDS, and William Mueller, DDS
Dermatology: Anna Bruckner, MD
Diabetes: Georgeanna Klingensmith, MD
Digital Health: Bonnie Offit, MD, Children's Hospital of Philadelphia
Ear, Nose, and Throat: Kenneth Chan, MD
Endocrinology: Michael Kappy, MD
Gastroenterology: David Brumbaugh, MD; Glenn Furuta, MD; Michael
   Narkewicz, MD; Jason Soden, MD; Judy Sondheimer, MD; Ronald Sokol, MD;
   and Sara Fidanza, RN, PNP
General Pediatrics: Steven Poole, MD; Stephen Berman, MD; Robert Brayden, MD;
   Brandi Freeman, MD; Allison Kempe, MD; Maya Bunik, MD; and Christopher
   Stille, MD
Hematology: Taru Hays, MD
Infectious Diseases: Jessica Cataldi, MD; Samuel Dominguez, MD; James K.
   Todd, MD; Ann-Christine Nyquist, MD; Mary Glode, MD; Mark Abzug, MD;
   Elizabeth McFarland, MD; Harley Rotbart, MD; and John Ogle, MD
Neonatology: Susan Niermeyer, MD; Elizabeth Thilo, MD; Mary Kohn, MD; and
   Adam Rosenberg, MD
Nephrology: Douglas Ford, MD
Neurology: Alan Seay, MD; Timothy Bernard, MD; Paul Moe, MD; Paul
   Levisohn, MD; and Julie Parsons, MD
Nutrition: Nancy Krebs, MD
Ophthalmology: Robert Enzenauer, MD, and Robert King, MD
Orthopedics: Frank Chang, MD, and Robert Eilert, MD

Pediatric Subspecialists: Children's Hospital Colorado, Aurora, CO *(Unless Otherwise Noted) (cont)*
Pulmonary Medicine: Monica Federico, MD; Gwendolyn Kerby, MD; and Scott Sagel, MD
Rheumatology: Roger Hollister, MD
Sports Medicine: Julie Wilson, MD
Toxicology: Richard Dart, MD, Medical Director, Rocky Mountain Poison Center, Denver, CO
Urology: Martin Koyle, MD

American Academy of Pediatrics Appointed Reviewers
Mark Corkings, MD, FAAP, Member, AAP Committee on Nutrition
Jesse Hackell, MD, FAAP, Chair, AAP Committee on Practice and Ambulatory Medicine
Leo Heitlinger, MD, FAAP, Chair, AAP Section on Gastroenterology, Hepatology, and Nutrition
Jack Swanson, MD, FAAP, Chair, AAP Committee on Practice and Ambulatory Medicine
Allan Lieberthal, MD, FAAP, Member, AAP Committee on Practice and Ambulatory Medicine
Nancy Krebs, MD, MS, FAAP, Member, AAP Committee on Nutrition
Jennifer Shu, MD, FAAP, Medical Editor, AAP HealthyChildren.org, official Web site for parents

Community Pediatricians
Justin Alvey, MD, Layton, UT
John Benbow, MD, Concord, NC
Barbara Brundage, MD, Derry, NH
Catherine Casey, MD, Arlington, VA
Thomas Foels, MD, Williamsville, NY
Cajsa Schumacher, MD, Albany, NY

Parent Reviewers
Lynnette Baer, Gayle Ebel, Candy Ergen, Carol Markley, Christina Podolak, Mary Schmitt, and Sandra Wilday; Littleton, CO
Nancy Gary, Doris Klein, and Sara Rotbart; Denver, CO
Elizabeth Berk; Concord, MA

Index

Page numbers in *italic* indicate a table.